EPIDEMIOLOGY OF COMMUNICABLE AND NON-COMMUNICABLE DISEASES - ATTRIBUTES OF LIFESTYLE AND NATURE ON HUMANKIND

Edited by **Fyson H. Kasenga**

Epidemiology of Communicable and Non-Communicable Diseases - Attributes of Lifestyle and Nature on Humankind

http://dx.doi.org/10.5772/61903
Edited by Fyson H. Kasenga

Contributors

Farouk Laabassi, Michał Polguj, Ludomir Stefańczyk, Mirosław Topol, Daynia Ballot, Tobias Chirwa, Tekin Guney, Aysun Senturk Yikilmaz, Imdat Dilek, João Mesquita, Fernando Esteves, Cármen Nóbrega, Carla Santos, António Monteiro, Rita Cruz, Helena Vala, Ana Cláudia Coelho, Tamer Hasan Hassan, Mohamed Badr, Usama El Safy, Mervat Hesham, Laila Sherief, Marwa Zakaria, Hachung Yoon

CBS, Edition **2017**

Published by InTech

Janeza Trdine 9, 51000 Rijeka, Croatia

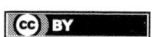
Notice

Publishing Process Manager Romina Rovan

Technical Editor SPi Global

Cover Designer InTech Design Team

Additional hard copies can be obtained from orders@intechopen.com

Epidemiology of Communicable and Non-Communicable Diseases - Attributes of Lifestyle and Nature on Humankind
Edited by Fyson H. Kasenga
p. cm.
Print ISBN 978-953-51-2740-6
Online ISBN 978-953-51-2741-3

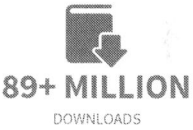
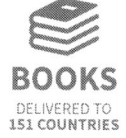
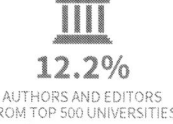
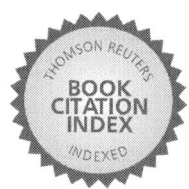

Contents

Preface VII

Section 1   Epidemiology of Communicable Diseases   1

Chapter 1   **Epidemiology and Investigation of Foot-and-Mouth Disease (FMD) in the Republic of Korea   3**
Hachung Yoon, Wooseog Jeong, Jida Choi, Yong Myung Kang and Hong Sik Park

Chapter 2   **Epidemiology of Equine Influenza Viruses   19**
Farouk Laabassi

Chapter 3   **Epidemiology and Emergence of Schmallenberg Virus Part 1: Origin, Transmission and Differential Diagnosis   33**
Fernando Esteves, João Rodrigo Mesquita, Cármen Nóbrega, Carla Santos, António Monteiro, Rita Cruz, Helena Vala and Ana Cláudia Coelho

Chapter 4   **Epidemiology and Emergence of Schmallenberg Virus Part 2: Pathogenesis and Risk of Viral Spread   57**
Fernando Esteves, João Rodrigo Mesquita, Cármen Nóbrega, Carla Santos, António Monteiro, Rita Cruz, Helena Vala and Ana Cláudia Coelho

Section 2   Epidemiology of Non-Communicable Disease   73

Chapter 5   **The Epidemiological, Morphological, and Clinical Aspects of the Aberrant Right Subclavian Artery (Arteria Lusoria)   75**
Michał Polguj, Ludomir Stefańczyk and Mirosław Topol

Chapter 6   **Factors Associated with Survival to Discharge of Newborns in a Middle-Income Country   87**
Daynia Elizabeth Ballot and Tobias Chirwa

Chapter 7 **Epidemiology of Vitamin B12 Deficiency 103**
Tekin Guney, Aysun Senturk Yikilmaz and Imdat Dilek

Chapter 8 **β-Thalassemia: Genotypes and Phenotypes 113**
Tamer Hassan, Mohamed Badr, Usama El Safy, Mervat Hesham,
Laila Sherief and Marwa Zakaria

Preface

Preventable diseases among cross-cultural communities are rampant, causing untold human suffering, and consequently untimely premature deaths occur particularly in poor-resource settings. These human sufferings, including deaths, can be reduced or avoided by applying routine principles of hygiene in individuals' lives as some of them are purely simple remedies, which are inexpensive, affordable, acceptable and easily accessible. Generally, it is an individual's responsibility to guard the different aspects of his or her own health, consequently resulting in a positive change in the lifestyle and good health-seeking behaviour.

It is in the view of the authors that the readers of this book will derive maximum benefits from it and act as change agents in their places of work and the communities they live or serve. It is evident that change is first enacted from within the mindset of an individual, then transmitted to families, groups and communities, and eventually the mindset of a nation can change creating an environment which is better for everybody to live in.

This book contains chapters discussing conditions or diseases that may not be common in the readers' area. Caution as such may never be underestimated considering the fact that we are living in a global village where one can never say 'this does not occur in my area' but rather question, does this occur in my community, why does it occur, who is affected, where and when does it occur and what can be done about it? These questions constitute what epidemiology is all about, and their precise and comprehensive answers can transform lives and help us have the right perceptions for the health challenges we face and accept the possibility of dealing with them directly. It is only when we can all jointly acknowledge and accept that 'this is our problem' as opposed to 'it is theirs' that this notion can help us deal with the 'epidemiology of communicable and non-communicable diseases: attributes of lifestyle and nature on humankind'.

Fyson H. Kasenga, PhD, MPH
Malawi Adventist University
Malamulo College of Health of Sciences
Makwasa, Malawi

Epidemiology of Communicable Diseases

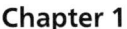

Epidemiology and Investigation of Foot-and-Mouth Disease (FMD) in the Republic of Korea

Hachung Yoon, Wooseog Jeong, Jida Choi,
Yong Myung Kang and Hong Sik Park

Additional information is available at the end of the chapter

http://dx.doi.org/10.5772/63975

Abstract

This chapter describes about the experience of dealing with FMD outbreaks in the Republic of Korea. We explain what is FMD, the concept of epidemiological investigation on outbreak sites of FMD, including the episode of detecting the index case for seven epidemics occurred since 2000, and information obtained from investigation in Korea. In any case, farmers' attitude (recognize clinical signs and report suspected cases) played the essential role in determining size and duration of epidemics. A rapid and correct diagnosis including clinical examination and laboratory test for confirmation is also important.

Keywords: foot-and-mouth disease (FMD), investigation, control measures, surveillance, Republic of Korea

1. Introduction

Foot-and-mouth disease (FMD) caused by virus infection of a small non-enveloped ribonucleic acid (RNA) virus belongs to family Picornaviridae, genus Aphthovirus. FMD virus affects Cloven-hoofed domestic animals including cattle, pig, sheep, goat, deer, boar, and wild animals. Due to its high contagiousness, FMD has a great potential for causing severe economic loss. There are seven immunologically distinct serotypes of FMD virus: O (Oise Valley), A (Allemand), C, Asia1, SAT (southern African territories)-1, SAT-2, SAT-3. According to the homogeneity of gene sequence of VP1 protein (approximately 639 base pairs, bps), the virus' topotype (concerns to the location) and lineage (concerns to the ancestor) are further catego-

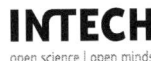

rized. RNA viruses show frequent spontaneous mutation, which results in emergence of new lineages. Phylogenetic analysis allows tracking the evolution and the origin of strains [1].

Clinical signs of FMD are characterized by vesicles in foot, mouth, and teats. Virus starts excreting 2 days before the appearance of clinical signs (4 days in case of milk), and antibody can be detected from 3-5 days after the appearance of clinical signs. High levels of antibodies are reached 2–4 days later and remained for many months. The virus disappears upon the appearance of antibody in most parts of the body. However, it continues to be detected exceptionally in laryngo-pharyngeal fluid. Antibodies to FMD virus are directed against structural proteins (SP) in the viral capsid and non-structural proteins (NSP) in the process of virus replication. SP antibodies are relatively serotype specific and induced by both vaccination and infection. Meanwhile, NSP antibodies are not serotype specific and induced by infection but rarely by non-purified vaccine also. SP antibodies usually start to appear approximately 3–4 days after the appearance of clinical signs, while 6–7 days in case of NSP antibodies [2, 3].

FMD occurs throughout the world, mainly in countries of Asia, Africa and parts of South America. It is the first disease for which the OIE (World Organisation for Animal Health) established an official list of free countries upon the science-based standards, guidelines and recommendations [4]. The Republic of Korea had been free from FMD without vaccination for the past 66 years, before a the outbreak of FMD in March 2000. In this chapter, epidemics of FMD in Korea from 2000 to 2015 are described together with their epidemiological character-istics.

2. Epidemics of FMD in Korea

Since 2000, Korea has experienced seven epidemics of FMD: March–April 2000, May–June 2002, January 2010, April–May 2010, November 2010–April 2011, July–August 2014, and December 2014–April 2015 [**Table 1** and **Figure 1**].

Year	2000	2002	2010				2014	
Month (Index region)			January (Pocheon)	April (Ganghwa)	November (Andong)		July (Euseong)	December (Jincheon)
Epidemic period	3.24–4.15 (23 days)	5.2–6.23 (53 days)	1.2–1.29 (28 days)	4.8–5.6 (29 days)	'10.11.28 –'11.4.21 (145 days)		7.23–8.6 (15 days)	'14.12.3 –'15.4.28 (147 days)
Number of outbreaks	15	16	6	11	153		3	185
Regions affected	6 counties in 3 provinces	4 counties in 2 provinces	2 counties in 1 province	4 counties in 4 provinces	75 counties in 11 provinces		3 counties in 2 provinces	33 counties in 7 provinces

Year	2000	2002	2010			2014	
Month (Index region)			January (Pocheon)	April (Ganghwa)	November (Andong)	July (Euseong)	December (Jincheon)
Serotype	O (Pan-Asia O_1)	O (Pan-Asia O_1)	A	O (SEA)	O (SEA)	O (SEA)	O (SEA)
Slaughter (No. of animals)	12,216 from 182 farms	160,155 from 162 farms	5,956 from 55 farms	49,874 from 395 farms	3,479,000 from 6,241 farms	2,009 from 3 farms	172,798 from 196 farms
Vaccination	Ring	None	None	None	Nationwide	Nationwide	Nationwide

Table 1. Epidemics of FMD in Korea from 2000 to 2015.

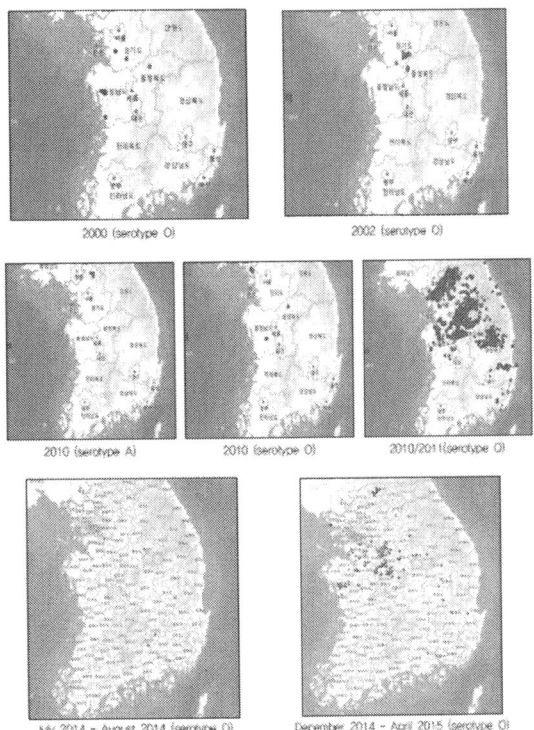

Figure 1. Distribution of outbreak farms of FMD in Korea from 2000 to 2015.

2.1. Epidemic in 2000

A suspected case was first reported from a dairy cattle farm in Paju, Gyeonggi-do, on 20 March 2000. Serotype O FMD virus was identified, which included in the Pan-Asian topotype. The route of virus introduction into Korea remains unclear. Fifteen outbreaks were reported until 15 April 2000. The outbreaks were concentrated in six counties of three provinces. There was one outbreak per county with the exception of one county, Hongseong, Chungcheongnam-do, from which 10 outbreaks were reported. All of the outbreaks in this epidemic involved cattle farm. A total of 2,216 cloven-hoofed animals of 182 farms were destroyed including all infected and neighbor farms within 500 m radius. Emergency vaccination (double-oil emulsion vaccines containing inactivated FMD virus strain O1 Manisa) of all susceptible animals within 3 km of radius of outbreak farms was performed. During the first round, 860,700 animals and 661,770 for the second booster round had been vaccinated by August 2000. All vaccinated animals except for soon to be slaughtered finishing pigs were indicated with ear marking either by punching holes (pigs) or by branding (cattle, goat, and deer). The animals have been registered and maintained by county offices to be directly transferred to designated slaughterhouses. Between first and second round of vaccinations, a total of 198,930 animals have been either slaughtered through a government buying out program or sent to the designated slaughterhouses. In the vaccinated zones, clinical inspections by field veterinarians as well as statistically designed serological surveillance were performed [5]. The country regained the previous status of FMD free country without vaccination from the OIE in September 2001.

2.2. Epidemic in 2002

On 2 May 2002, a suspect case with vesicles on the nose, tongue, hoof and teat, deletion of hooves, and high mortality in piglets was reported at a pig farm located in Anseong, Gyeonggi-do. The second case was reported the next day at a pig farm in Jincheon, Chungcheongbuk-do. Serotype O FMD was confirmed on a total of 16 farms (15 pig farms and one cattle farm). It was concluded that the use of vaccines was not advisable for this epidemic. The following facts explain the reasons: The outbreaks were in intensive pig farming areas and some surrounding farms would already likely be infected; period required for pigs to gain immunity is 2–3 weeks, during which they would still be vulnerable to infection; the use of vaccination would prolong the required period to regain FMD free status; there was a risk of spread by vaccination teams; and vaccination would hinder the effectiveness of surveillance, making it difficult to detect any new FMD cases. Most of all, the epidemic was not spreading out of control [6].

2.3. Epidemic in January 2010

A private veterinarian notified early symptoms indicative of FMD such as loss of appetite and hyper-salivation on a dairy cattle farm in Pocheon, Gyeonggi-do, on 2 January 2010. Local veterinary service visited the farm, but lack of FMD-specific lesions at that time interfered a proper sampling for laboratory test. The farm was placed under close observation. On 6 January, FMD-specific lesions including erosion and ulcer in oral cavity and nasal passage, as well as ulcer and crust on teats, were observed. FMD virus serotype A was confirmed. All of six cases in cattle farm in this epidemic were detected within 3.8 km radius from the first outbreak farm [7].

2.4. Epidemic in April to May 2010

An outbreak of FMD serotype O was confirmed on April 9, following the previous day's notification of vesicles in the mouth and teats from a Hanwoo (Korean native beef cattle) farm in Ganghwa county of Incheon metropolis. As the second to fifth outbreaks, all occurred in the adjacent area, control measures including preemptive culling for all susceptible livestock in the protection zones within 3 km, were focused to prevent further spread of FMD. Extensive disinfection was carried out passing through two bridges connecting the Ganghwa Island to the mainland. Despite these collective efforts, on 21 April, a suspected case was reported at a pig farm located 135 km away from the previous outbreak area. Additional two outbreaks occurred in the latter area, Cheongyang, Chungcheongnam-do, by 6 May. Comparison of the VP1 region of FMD viruses isolated from the infected farms showed 99.68–100% homology, suggesting that all of 11 outbreaks were from a same origin [7].

2.5. Epidemic in November 2010 to April 2011

FMD occurred three times in 2010 (January, April, and November). The first case of the third epidemic was reported on 28 November 2010, from one of the five pig farms in a complex in Andong, Gyeongsangbuk-do. When officers of national veterinary services arrived in the farm, approximately 700 dead piglets were piled up in the farm yard. They found out that FMD was already widespread in all five piggeries. The oldest lesion was observed at the innermost farm. Until 21 April 2011, for 145 days, FMD outbreaks were confirmed in 153 farms raising cattle, pigs, goats, or deer in 75 counties of 11 provinces. Serotype O SEA topotype (Mya-98 lineage) was isolated. Phylogenetic analysis showed nucleotide differences more or less 1.0% among FMD virus of outbreak farms. In early December 2010, FMD broke out primarily on Hanwoo (Korean native beef cattle) farms around the index case in Andong. However, on 14 December, two pig farms in Yeoncheon and Yangju in northern Gyeonggi-do, belonged to the same owner, also reported FMD suspected animals. The nationwide spread of FMD was imminent. The epidemic continued until April of the next year [8]. The status of an FMD-free country with vaccination was recognized by the OIE on 27 May 2014, 3 years after the last cases of the epidemics in April 2011. The approval was obtained after the review of the report, submitted on October 2013, which verified the non-circulation of FMD virus for more than a year based on a test of non-structural protein (NSP) antibodies in vaccinated animals.

Implementation of a vaccine containing inactivated O1 Manisa strain (monovalent) was urgently implemented. Injections were first administered on 25 December 2010, to cattle near the outbreak areas. Vaccination of pigs was first implemented on 6 January 2011. The program was gradually extended, and all cattle and pigs in Korea were subject to injection from 15 January 2011. The second set of injections was started on 23 January in cattle and 3 February in pigs, respectively, and completed by 26 February. In the case of pigs, the outbreak decreased remarkably 3 weeks after primary vaccination, while in the case of cattle, it decreased after 2 weeks. From 3 March, additional vaccination was implemented to animals born without maternal antibodies because they were born before the beginning of vaccination, and pigs at 3–4 weeks before delivery. And deer and goats were also added to the vaccine object. Since September 2011, it was mandatory for all cloven-hoofed animals to be implemented with trivalent (O, A, Asia 1) vaccination by 6-month interval. Before nationwide vaccination, all animals in the outbreak farm were stamped out. However, after 27 January 2011, when the nationwide vaccination was successfully completed, only animals showing symptoms or a positive reaction were stamped out [8].

2.6. Epidemic in July to August 2014

On 23 July 2014, the suspected animals were reported from 1 pig farm with 1,500 animals in Euseong, Gyeongsangbuk-do. The presence of FMD virus was confirmed in the next morning. Clinical signs appeared in unvaccinated animals in that farm. Subsequently, FMD was diagnosed in two more farms by 6 August 2014 [9].

2.7. Epidemic in December 2014 to April 2015

After 4 months, on 3 December 2014, a veterinarian of a farm with 15,884 animals in Jincheon, Chungcheongbuk-do, observed vesicles and ataxia in 30 pigs and reported the same to the county office. FMD was confirmed on the next day. During the next 147 days, until 28 April 2015, 180 pig farms and 5 cattle farms were confirmed with FMD [9].

3. On farm investigation

3.1. Regulation associated to investigation

In the Republic of Korea, in case of FMD outbreak, control measures are implemented based on the investigation of outbreak epidemiology. Both investigation and control measures were stipulated by the Act on the Prevention of Contagious Animal Diseases, the FMD Control Guidelines, and the standard operation procedure for FMD. These regulations include notification of suspected cases, movement control, stamping-out, disinfection, regular and emergency vaccination, import quarantine, disposal, compensation, and penalties [8, 9].

3.2. Principle of investigation

A smart investigation on the epidemiology of outbreak is crucial in order to implement control measures in case of confirming FMD. In case of FMD outbreak, the veterinary epidemiology division of the Animal and Plant Quarantine Agency (QIA) took overall responsibility for the epidemiological investigation throughout Korea. Field investigation and contact tracing were performed for each outbreak farm and putative dangerous contacts. All movements in-and-out associated with animals, people, vehicles, and materials were investigated for each farm for at least 21-day period (14 days in case of vaccination) immediately before the outbreak date. Then, the forward-and-backward tracings, which list up all the places visited before and after being at the outbreak farm, were performed for each visitor, resident, and worker related to the farm [10].

3.3. Example of field investigation in Korea

A template to guide epidemiological investigation on the outbreak site is is prepared. The investigation process includes three steps: confirming infection, estimating date of first infection and determining mode of introduction. Below is example of investigation on FMD outbreak in Korea.

3.3.1. Confirming infection

FMD suspected animals were reported from a pig farm with 1,552 pigs in two houses located adjacent to buildings of pork-processing plant, on 2 June 2002. FMD outbreak in this farm was confirmed on 3 June, based on serological and virological tests.

3.3.2. Estimating date of first infection

In the late evening of 1 June, one of the farm workers notified "something abnormal on the hooves of the growing pigs to the owner. O the next morning, upon reporting of the owner, staffs of QIA (it was named National Veterinary Research and Quarantine Service, NVRQS, at that time) visited the site and observed intact vesicles (nasal plane, oral cavity, and coronary band), ruptured vesicles (coronary band), lameness, anorexia, and fever on nine animals examined in detail. Based on the number of animals with clinical signs and the age of the oldest lesion, the first clinical sign was estimated to have been developed since 7 days. Considering the incubation time of 4 days (a range of 2–14 days), FMD virus infection in this herd was the most likely to start on on 22 May (12 May at the earliest to 24 May at the latest)s.

3.3.3. Determining mode of introduction

Through field investigation and tracing, a total of 229 farms had contacts with this outbreak farm during 21-day period before the notification, either via people or vehicles visited to this farm or via slaughterhouse to which pigs were sent from this farm. No pigs had been introduced onto this farm. Preemptive slaughter was undertaken on three farms having epidemiological associations: One farm had dangerous contact such as sharing a common pig-transport truck, and the other two were located within 3-km distance from the outbreak farm.

A direct link was identified between this farm, reported on 2 June and the index farm, reported on 2 May. There was a person (man) worked at the neighboring pork-processing plant on a part-time basis, which was operated by the same owner with the outbreak farm. He has also participated in the culling operations on the index farm during three consecutive days from 3 May. He drove his car to the local animal health service then transported to the slaughter site, in wearing a T-shirt, a pair of blue jeans, and a pair of boots. At the slaughter site, disposable work-suit and boot covers were provided. After completing the operation, he cleaned himself at a public bath together with other workers. Then, he put new underwear and shirts provided by the local government. But, he put again the same trouser that he wore in working because he had no spare one. While he took a bath, his jean was wrapped in a vinyl bag after being sprayed disinfectant. He returned back home by his own car in which no disinfection measures were implemented. He worked at the port-processing plant for three or four occasions, starting on 8 May. FMD virus was probably transmitted by this person considering that the index farm, on which 330 (4.0%) of 8,302 pigs showed clinical signs or died at the time of culling, was heavily contaminated at the time of culling. FMD virus must survive in environment such as interior of his car, and transmitted to the pork-processing plant and adjacent pig houses during 17 days of interval between the completion of culling (5 May) and the most likely date of first infection (22 April) [10].

4. Clinical signs

By carrying out epidemiological investigation, we can estimate how long has the disease been on the farm, where did the disease come from, and where the disease might have spread to. To establish a likely time period of infection dynamics took place in animals of the farm, aging clinical lesions is important. Looking for the oldest lesions allows identifying the time of first infection in the herd. Clinical examination starts by taking history about type and time of clinical signs and affected animals from the farmer. Then, the animals from a distance to see general demeanor, salivation, lameness, or ataxia were observed. When we examine the individual animal, check the mouth (especially in cattle) then the feet (in pigs) in order.

The clinical signs of FMD were the most clearly manifested in pigs followed by dairy cattle comparing to other species. In the epidemic of 2010/2011, only 2.6% of the dairy cattle farms and 1.9% of the pig farms were subclinically infected, while no clinical signs of FMD was observed in 10-20% of the outbreak farms with beef cattle, deer, or goats. For beef cattle, the number of farms with ulcers (n = 408, 28.6%) was higher than that showing vesicles (n = 316, 22.2%). For dairy cattle, on the contrary, vesicles (n = 166, 32.6%) were more frequent than ulcers (n = 107, 21.0%) in dairy cattle farms. In 58.9% of the pig farms, vesicle was the most dominant sign of FMD. In pigs, more severe signs, such as lameness or ataxia (14.6%) and shedding of claws (4.6%), were also distinctively shown. Another clinical characteristic observed in the 2010/2011 FMD epidemic was sudden death of suckling piglets, which was observed in 21.2% of pig farms. The average age of the oldest lesion in an outbreak farm was higher in the vaccinated than the non-vaccinated in cattle, while it was higher in non-vaccinated in pigs. Considering that vaccination was firstly performed on cattle then on pigs, and the outbreaks continued only in pig farms at the later phase of the epidemic, difference of lesions' age between cattle and pig at detecting seemed mainly associated with farmers' attention and recognition [11].

In the epidemic of 2014/2015, any clinical signs of FMD were observed in all of the 185 outbreak farms. Vesicles, which were observed 65.0% of the outbreak pig farms, were the most prominent clinical signs, followed by lameness (43.9%), ataxia (38.9%), and hemorrhage in hooves (25.0%) [9].

5. Detection of outbreak farms

Detection of outbreak farm signifies the start of implementing control measures by animal health service. Large number of outbreak farms in the epidemics of 2010/2011 and 2014/2015 were attributed to the late detection of the infection, and FMD virus was already spread out at the time of confirming the index case [8, 9].

5.1. Delayed detection

In case of the 2010/2011 epidemic, implementation of control measures was delayed due to inappropriate diagnosis. When the first suspected case was reported on 23 November 2010, the NSP antibody test was conducted on the clinically suspected animals which had not yet developed NSP antibody, and negative results were drawn. Three days later, when the farmer notified the abnormalities for the second time, antibody test confirmed negative results again. Antibodies can be detected by enzyme-linked immunosorbent assay(ELISA) test from 3–5 days after appearing clinical signs of FMD. Finally, FMD was confirmed in isolating virus through reverse transcription-polymerase chain reaction (RT-PCR) by the QIA from the specimen taken on 28 November [12].

5.2. Early detection

On the contrary, prompt diagnosis contributed to the reduction of disease spread in the epidemic of 2002. From 9 May, 1 week after the confirmation of the first case, pen-side antigen test, which can detect FMD virus in vesicular fluids, was used for FMD suspect cases. This test enabled confirmation of infection to be made on the farm in about 20 min. Stamping out was implemented based on clinical examination (observing vesicles in most cases) and the pen-side antigen test results even before laboratory confirmation was made in some cases. During this epidemic, 13 of the 16 outbreak farms were culled within 24 h of diagnosis, which was an important factor in reducing the spread of the disease [6].

5.3. Probability of detection

The probability of early detection was the highest for pig farms, followed by dairy and beef cattle farms, and small ruminant farms in the case of the 2010/2011 epidemic. Almost 90% of the infected farms were detected by Day 11 of post-infection for pig farms, by Day 13 for both dairy and beef cattle farms, and by Day 21 for small ruminant farms. As far as concerned to the detection delay, that was time passed prior to the detection of FMD infection on a farm (average ± standard deviation), was 8.1 ± 3.1 days. The detection delays were shortest for pig farms (7.1 ± 2.5 days) and longest for deer farms where a large variation was also observed (14.4 ± 8.1 days) [13].

6. Epidemiological characteristics of FMD epidemics

Throughout the seven epidemics occurred since 2000, pig and cattle were the main species affected by FMD outbreak. The main factors of virus transmission were associated with the movement of vehicles, behaviors of people, and distribution of materials rather than movement of animals. Epidemics started in winter were usually long and large. The cold and dry winter climate in Korea made favorable condition for surviving FMD virus. In addition, low temperature during the winter might have preserved FMD virus for longer periods. Disinfecting farms, vehicles, and tools wasn't effective because the low temperature let disinfectants freeze. The hygiene status of livestock farms remained poor and animal disease could spread widely and rapidly. Epidemics of the 2010/2011 and 2014/2015 were the cases.

6.1. Characteristics of epidemic in 2002

The index case of the 2002 epidemic was notified on 2 May 2002. The next day, on 3 May, the second outbreak was notified at a pig farm in 25 km away from the index case. Based on the epidemiological investigation, FMD virus was probably spread from the index case to the second outbreak farm by a salesperson of a veterinary pharmaceutical company. Subsequently developed two spatial clusters centered of these farms and all known outbreak farms were encompassed except for one case. Genetic analysis of virus isolates from all of 15 outbreak farms, except for one from which no viral isolate was obtained, suggested that they had originated from a single common source. Herd serial interval of disease transmission at farm level was 8–9 (average ± standard deviation, 9.1 ± 2.0, median 8.5) days, and the transmission was extended into five generations. Eight farms were already infected before detecting the index case. A study on simulation modeling on various control strategy for the epidemic in 2002 suggested that the prompt implementation of control measures is the most effective in reducing both size and duration of future outbreaks [14].

6.2. Characteristics of epidemic in January 2010

The index case farm for the epidemic of January 2010 employed a foreigner, entered Korea on October 2009, as a farm hand. Disinfection or other biosecurity measures had not been taken before starting work on that farm. Furthermore, a parcel was delivered to the person above-mentioned from his country on November 2009. In 2009, countries in northeast Asia had numerous outbreaks reported of FMD serotype A. Considering these findings, employment of a foreign worker in the first outbreak farm was identified as a possible route of virus introduction into Korea. FMD virus was subsequently transmitted to other farms through local veterinarian's examination, farmers' meeting, and farm owner's visit to the infected area [15]. The honest report of the local veterinarian his visiting places allowed to detect potential infections in early stage then promptly implement control measures. Unlikely to other epidemics during winter, heavy snow of early January 2010 in the outbreak area helped to restrict moving vehicles. So the spread of virus could be minimized.

6.3. Characteristics of epidemic in April to May 2010

Investigation for the epidemic from April to May 2010 identified possible routes of between-farm transmission were mostly associated with livestock related vehicles including contaminated feed-delivery vehicles, artificial inseminators, and delivery of veterinary pharmaceutics, total mixed ration (TMR) feed. Meetings of livestock-related people, visits to contaminated regions, vehicle movements, sales agents of animal feed companies, and participants of livestock culling seemed also contributed [15].

6.4. Characteristics of epidemic in November 2010 to April 2011

In the epidemic from November 2010 to April 2011, the routes of FMD virus introduction and their estimated frequencies for the 152 subsequent outbreaks except for the index case pig-farming complex were visitors (105, 69.1%), farmers (23, 15.1%), local spread (18, 11.8%), and delivered materials (6, 3.9%). Six outbreak farms, for which virus pathway was attributed to visitors, were associated with treatment or manipulation of artificial insemination, and 14 outbreaks were due to vehicles transporting live animals. The initial contributing factor of the 2010/2011 nationwide FMD epidemic was the regional feature of Andong, Gyeongsangbuk-do, where the residents were closely related to each other. During the epidemic, the frequent contacts might help the virus spread rapidly out to adjacent areas. The main cause of the long-distance virus' spread to the northern Gyeonggi-do was presumed to be related to the transport of pig manure to be used to installation test of a manure treatment machine. On 17 November 2010, pig manure from the pig complex in Andong was sent to the developer of the manure drying machine in Paju, Gyeonggi-do. The FMD virus already had been spread to nearby farms in the northern Gyeonggi-do area before any preventive measure was taken. The first outbreak in northern Gyeonggi-do was occurred on the same day of 14 December 2010 in two farming sites with a large number of pigs, operated by a same owner. Many farms raising cattle or pigs existed nearby, and shared road. Through traffic in front of the farms, the virus spread quickly to nearby areas. The FMD outbreak in the densely located big farms led to difficulties in taking emergency control measures due to the lack of burial sites and slaughter personnel. These caused FMD spread widely [8].

6.5. Characteristics of epidemic in December 2014 to April 2015

During the outbreak of December 2014 to April 2015, FMD virus was introduced into 185 outbreak farms mostly by vehicles (143 cases, 78.9%), people (23 cases, 10.8%), local spread (16 cases, 8.6%), and movement of animals (3 cases, 1.6%) in the descending order. The pathways for spreading the virus to farms in other counties included (1) visits by vehicles (or drivers) contaminated at abattoirs, (2) vehicles (or drivers) visiting numerous farms, (3) distribution of infected animals to other farms, (4) distribution of feed from a factory affiliated to a large company to farms in various provinces, and (5) operation of two or more farms located in different provinces by one person (or members of the same family or an affiliated company). Meanwhile, delivery of veterinary pharmaceuticals, delivery of semen for artificial insemination, and transport of manure were associated with transmission within the same county or province. Vehicles and people, responsible for the introduction of FMD virus into farms, were contaminated at abattoirs (75 cases, 40.5%); livestock facilities (93 cases, 50.3%), including feed factories (17 cases, 9.7%); previous outbreak farms (67 cases, 36.2%); and infected areas (24 cases, 13.0%). FMD outbreaks continued for a long time since December 2014 because of the following reasons: (1) The virus continued to replicate among farms where animals were partially slaughtered; (2) the number of subsequent outbreak farms was inversely related to the proportion of FMD vaccine antibodies at county level; (3) control measures were not implemented at proper times Because farmers were reluctant to report suspected cases; and (4) outbreaks began in December, at the beginning of winter, during which the conditions were favorable for virus survival [9].

7. Economic Impacts of FMD outbreaks

The cost of each epidemic varied from 26 billion Korean won (KRW, approximately US$ 23.6 million) at the lowest to 2044 billion KRW (US$ 1.9 billion) at the highest. The cost was the highest for the 2000 epidemic, to which vaccination to slaughter policy was implemented to control outbreaks of 15 cattle farms. Mean cost attributed to one outbreak cattle farm was 18.2 billion KRW. In 2002, January 2010 and April to May 2010 epidemics with slaughter without vaccination costed 6.6 billion KRW, 4.4 billion KRW, and 9.2 billion KRW, respectively. Then, vaccination-to-live policy dragged the lowest costs of 0.5 billion for the 2010/2011 and 0.3 billion for the 2014/2015 epidemic [16].

The highest cost of an outbreak of FMD reached in cattle farms. Average costs per infected premises were 7.0 billion KRW for cattle farms (95% confidence interval, CI = 4.72–9.28), 1.38 billion KRW for pig farms (95% CI = 0.88–1.87), 0.11 billion KRW for deer [16].

8. Surveillance

The surveillance system consists of passive epidemiological surveillance for investigating reported disease and active epidemiological surveillance that involves serological surveillance. The latter can be further divided into statistically designed surveillance and purposive surveillance focusing on targeted samples within host populations. On the other hand, clinical surveillance included clinical inspection And telephone calls. Emergency vaccination was launched in end of December, the middle of the 2010/2011 epidemic. And Only animals with positive reaction or showing clinical signs of FMD were slaughtered. The NSP antibody test on the outbreak farm was conducted together with clinical inspection at 3 weeks after the partial slaughter. The NSP antibody tests were conducted on all cattle, deer, and goats. In pig farms, all sows and three fattening pigs per pen were subjected to be tested. This test was aiming at getting rid of movement restriction on the outbreak farm. After 26 March 2011, the effective preventive measures at the site: clinical, serological (16 animals per farm), and environmental antigen tests were conducted on cattle, deer, and goats, and clinical examination and environmental antigen test were conducted on pigs.

Post-vaccination seroprevalence must be examined on vaccinated animals. This can be performed using commercial diagnostic kits. Sera are collected from farms and slaughter-houses. Purpose of this serological surveillance is to assure the OIE Code for FMD states that all vaccinated animals should develop at least 80% protective immunity to be recognized as a FMD-free country with vaccination [12].

9. Data management

Korea Animal Health Integrated System (KAHIS) is in operation since January 2013. This system contains all data concerning livestock and animal health in Korea. Data on farm (owner, geolocation, farm type, animals), livestock-related facilities (slaughter house, feed factory or feed distribution center, manured disposal plant, livestock market, veterinary clinics, veterinary pharmaceutical agencies, semen for artificial insemination distribution center, etc.) and vehicles transporting (animals, raw milk, eggs, veterinary pharmaceutics, feed, feces, manure, rice husks) and for the use of personnel (veterinarian, artificial inseminator, consultant, specimen taking and control, machine mender) are available. When a vehicle visits farm or livestock-related facility, the receiver installed on the site recognized the signal from the geographical positioning system (GPS) tracking device attached to the vehicle. A real time inquiry can be made on data of visit record both on the aspects of farm and vehicles. In addition, all the pathway of a vehicle can be traced. This web-based system is available at http://www.kahis.go.kr [17].

10. Conclusion

During the epidemic of 2010/2011, FMD virus had already widely spread before detecting the index case and it induced unprecedentedly large number of outbreak. The animal health service of Korea failed to respond timey and adequately due to lack of experience of controlling a massive epidemic of FMD with emergency vaccination to live. In the same manner, another big epidemic was occurred in 2014/2015 under routine vaccination.

As mentioned in the example of the 2002 epidemic, prompt implementation of control measures (e.g. removal of virus reservoirs), immediately after an early detection is the most effective to control FMD. The key determinant of the early detection is the report. In reality, an immediate report subsequent to recognizing abnormality is the collaboration with local veterinarians, related industries and animal health services. And this collaboration can be achieved upon proper education.

Author details

Hachung Yoon*, Wooseog Jeong, Jida Choi, Yong Myung Kang and Hong Sik Park

*Address all correspondence to: heleney@korea.kr

Animal and Plant Quarantine Agency, Gimcheon, Gyeongsangbuk-do, Republic of Korea

References

[1] Alexandersen S, Zhang Z, Donaldson AI, Garland AJM. The pathogenesis and diagnosis of foot-and-mouth disease. J Comp Path. 2003;129:1–36.

[2] Kitching RP. Clinical variation in foot and mouth disease: cattle. Rev Sci Tech Off Int Epiz. 2002;21(3):499–504.

[3] Kitching RP. Clinical variation in foot and mouth disease: pigs. Rev Sci Tech Off Int Epiz. 2002;21(3):513–518.

[4] OIE. About FMD. Foot and mouth disease Portal [Internet]. 2016; Available from: http://www.oie.int/animal-health-in-the-world/fmd-portal/about-fmd/ [Accessed:2016-03-21]

[5] Joo YS, An SH, Kim OK, Lubroth J, Sur JH. Foot-and-mouth disease eradication efforts in the Republic of Korea. Can J Vet Res. 2002;66(2):122–124.

[6] Wee SH, Yoon H, More SJ, Nam HM, Moon OK, Jung JM, Kim SJ, Kim CH, Lee ES, Park CK, Hwang IJ. Epidemiological characteristics of the 2002 outbreak of foot-and-mouth disease in the Republic of Korea. Transbound Emerg Dis. 2008;55(8):360–368.

[7] Park JH, Lee KN, Ko YJ, Kim SM, Lee HS, Shin YK, Sohn HJ, Park JY, Yeh JY, Lee YH, Kim MJ, Joo YS, Yoon H, Yoon SS, Cho IS, Kim BH. Control of foot-and-mouth disease during 2010–2011 epidemic, South Korea. Emerg Infect Dis. 2013;19(4):655–659.

[8] Yoon H, Yoon SS, Kim YJ, Moon OK, Wee SH, Joo YS, Kim B. Epidemiology of the foot-and-mouth disease serotype O epidemic of November 2010 to April 2011 in the Republic of Korea. Transbound Emerg Dis. 2015;62:252–263.

[9] Animal and Plant Quarantine Agency. 2014/2015 Epidemiological investigation analysis report on foot-and-mouth disease in the Republic of Korea, Anyang. QIA. 2014.

[10] Wee SH, Nam HM, Moon Ok, Yoon H, Park JY, More SJ. Using field-based epidemiological methods to investigate FMD outbreaks: An example from the 2002 outbreaks in Korea. Transbound Emerg Dis. 2008;55:404–410.

[11] Yoon H, Yoon SS, Wee SH, Kim YJ, Kim B. Clinical manifestation of foot-and-mouth disease during the 2010/2011 epidemic in the Republic of Korea. Transbound Emerg Dis. 2012;59(6):517–525.

[12] Animal, Plant and Fisheries Quarantine and Inspection Agency (QIA). Committee of epidemiological investigation. Report of epidemiological investigation on the 2010/2011 epidemic of FMD, Anyang. 2011.

[13] Yoon H, Yoon SS, Kim H, Kim YJ, Kim B, Wee SH. Estimation of the infection window for the 2010/2011 Korean foot-and-mouth disease outbreak. Osong Public Health Res Perspect. 2013;4(3):127–1312.

[14] Yoon H, Wee SH, Stevenson MA, O'Leary B, Morris RS, Hwang IJ, Park CK. Simulation analyses to evaluate alternative control strategies for the 2002 foot-and-mouth disease outbreak in the Republic of Korea. Prev Vet Med. 2006;74:212–225.

[15] Animal, Plant and Fisheries Quarantine and Inspection Agency (QIA). Committee of epidemiological investigation. Report of epidemiological investigation on the 2010 epidemic of FMD, Anyang. 2010.

[16] Kim H, Yoon H, Moon OK, Han JH, Lee K, Jeong W, Choi J, Cho YM, Kang YM, Ahn HY, Kim DS, Carpenter TE. Direct costs of five foot-and-mouth disease epidemics in the Republic of Korea, from 2000 to 2011. J Prev Vet Med. 2013;37(4):163–168. doi: 10.13041/jpvm.2013.37.4.163

[17] Animal and Plant Quarantine Agency. Korea Animal Health Integrated System. 2013. Available from: http://www.kahis.go.kr [Accessed:2016-03-21].

Chapter 2

Epidemiology of Equine Influenza Viruses

Farouk Laabassi

Additional information is available at the end of the chapter

http://dx.doi.org/10.5772/64588

Abstract

The equine influenza virus (EIV) is a major pathogen of respiratory diseases in horses, donkeys and mules. Equine influenza (EI) is characterized by a very rapid spread and remains a disease with high economic stakes for the equine industry. A large-scale outbreak caused by equine influenza virus of the H3N8 subtype has occurred in each decade since an H3N8 was first isolated from horses in 1963. Each epidemic, and some minor outbreaks, has influenced equine influenza surveillance and vaccination policies in the world. The use of the molecular tools is of a high interest in epidemiology. The interest of the association of these techniques and the classical epidemiological analyses will be illustrated by taking the example of equine influenza viruses. The determination and the comparison of the nucleotide sequences allow to characterize the virus strains more precisely than the classical methods and are useful to analyze the evolution of the equine influenza viruses. These methods are also useful to select the relevant strains that will be used in the vaccines. The possible reasons for the infection of horses despite intensive vaccination are currently being investigated and may shed new light on the epidemiology of equine influenza.

Keywords: equine influenza virus, epidemiology, pathogen, vaccination, vaccine strains selection

1. Introduction

Equine influenza (EI) is an important equine respiratory pathogen and a high-priority disease for the equine industry globally. It is highly contagious and spreads rapidly in horse population by direct contact; clinical signs associated with the infection are characterized by pyrexia, dyspnoea, dry hacking cough and serous nasal discharge that can become mucopurulent in the case of secondary bacterial infections [1]. The causative agent, equine influenza virus (EIV), has a global distribution; it is endemic in many countries and there are occasional incursions in

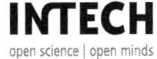

Japan, South Africa and Hong Kong, with only Australia, New Zealand and Iceland being considered free.

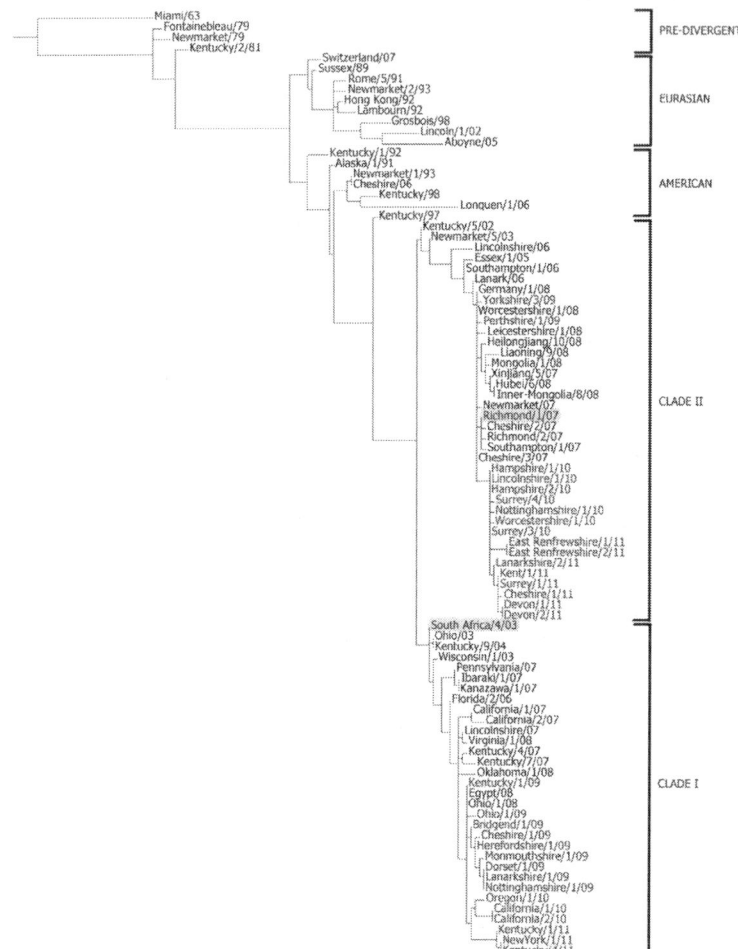

Figure 1. Phylogenetic analysis of the HA1 nucleotide sequences encoded by 90 EIV, subtype H3N8 isolated since 1963 and prototype strains of the different lineages and clades. Sequences are coloured by date of isolation for the years 2011 (red), 2010 (green) and 2009 (blue), with older strains in black. Current OIE recommended vaccine strains are highlighted in yellow [1].

EIV is belonging to the family of the *Orthomyxoviridae*, genus *Influenzavirus*, type A and is a major cause of respiratory diseases in horses. Only two antigenic subtypes of EIV (H7N7 and H3N8) have been isolated from horses, although highly pathogenic avian influenza virus

(H5N1) was isolated from donkeys in Egypt [2]. The equine H7N7 virus first isolated in Prague (Czechoslovakia) in 1956 [3] and has not been isolated in horses since 1979 [4], but serological evidence for its circulation in unvaccinated horses has been recorded at the end of the 1980s in India [5] and at the beginning of the 1990s in Croatia and USA [6, 7]. Since then, the equine H3N8 virus, first isolated in 1963 after an important outbreak in Miami (Florida, USA) [8], has persisted [9, 10] and only has been isolated from sick horses [11–15]. Phylogenetic studies have shown that H3N8 virus evolved in the late 1980s, into the American and the Eurasian lineages [16]. The Eurasian lineage strains, were almost exclusively isolated from horses in Europe and Asia, represented by Newmarket/2/93, continue to form a single clade, but have rarely been isolated in recent years [17]. The American lineage strains, were predominantly isolated from horses on the continent of America, further evolved into three sublineages, South American, Kentucky and Florida [18]. The original American lineage strains, represented by Newmarket/1/93 and Kentucky/1994, have not been completely superseded, with isolations of strains from this clade in the United Kingdom [17] and Chile [19] in 2006. The evolution of the Florida sublineage resulted in the emergence of two groups of viruses that differ in their HA sequences referred as Clade 1 viruses that have been isolated in North America since 2003 (e.g. Ohio/2003) and are distinct from the Florida Clade 2 strains that spread to Europe (Newmarket/5/03) [17]. Clade 1 viruses predominate on the American continent; nevertheless, they have caused large outbreaks in Africa, Asia, Australia, Europe and South America [20–27]. Similarly, Clade 2 viruses predominate in Europe but also have been isolated in Asia and North Africa [15, 28–32]. The phylogenetic analysis points to sporadic incursions of virus from North America into Europe and other regions, as happened around 1993 and 2003, followed by a period of more localized divergent evolution (**Figure 1**).

The use of the molecular tools is of a high interest in epidemiology. The interest of the association of these techniques and the classical epidemiological analyses will be illustrated by considering the example of equine influenza viruses. The determination and the comparison of the nucleotide sequences allow to characterize the virus strains more precisely than the classical methods and are useful to analyze the evolution of the equine influenza viruses. These methods are also useful to select the relevant strains that will be used in the vaccines. The possible reasons for the infection of horses despite intensive vaccination are currently being investigated and may shed new light on the epidemiology of equine influenza [33].

Influenza is a classic example of a (re-)emerging infection. Vaccines against influenza have been used in man since the 1940s [34] and became available for use in horses 20 years later. However, the existence of a reservoir of virus in aquatic birds and the highly variable nature of the virus mean that influenza defies worldwide eradication. The prevention and control of influenza are closely related measures of vaccination and livestock management. Vaccination is to date the most average usual to limit the spread of the virus in the horse population. Vaccines against equine influenza must contain subtypes and, inside thereof, the antigenic variants circulating in the horse population. Every year, the expert surveillance panel (ESP) of the World Organization for Animal Health (OIE) recommends influenza virus strains to be contained equine vaccines. The fact that H7N7 viruses and Eurasian H3N8 viruses are no longer required, current vaccines should include the antigenic variants of viruses representing each of Clades 1 and 2 of the Florida sublineage. The Clade 1 is represented by A/equine/South Africa/4/2003-like or A/equine/Ohio/2003-like viruses. The Clade 2 is represented by A/equine/Richmond/1/2007-like viruses.

2. Epidemiology

2.1. Incubation period

EI is characterized by an incubation period of 5 days a maximum and an infective period of 14 days. An incubation period of 2–3 days has been observed in susceptible horse populations during severe epidemics in the field. In naive horses, the incubation period can be less than 24 h [35] and virus excretion may persist for 7–10 days [36]. Most shedding occurs in the early stages of clinical disease when coughing is most pronounced. In partially immune horses showing no clinical signs or mild clinical signs, virus shedding may occur.

2.2. Interspecies transmission of equine influenza viruses

There are three types of influenza viruses: A, B and C, but only the first has a very high propensity to crossing species barrier, the two others being found almost exclusively in humans. Influenza A viruses met in several species including birds, humans, swine, horses, marine mammals and dogs. Only a restricted number of sub-type combinations have become established in mammalian species (H7N7 and H3N8 in horses; H1N1, H3N2 and H2N2 in humans) [37]. Recently, two distinct lineages (H17N10 and H18N11) of influenza A virus have been derived from bats. This discovery provided novel insights into the origin and evolution of influenza A viruses beyond the predominant hypothesis of waterfowls/shorebirds as the primary natural reservoir.

The equine influenza virus infects horses and other equids (such as donkeys, mules and zebras) can, but rarely affects other species (such as dogs) [38]. Studies have shown that the H3N8 sub-type was introduced into horses a long time ago and the lack of exchange of virus genes between the equine viruses and viruses from other species [39] led to the suggestion that horses may be a 'dead-end' host. However, in Florida (US) at the beginning of 2004, equine influenza virus has been associated with outbreaks of respiratory disease in dogs (primarily but not exclusively, greyhounds) in North America, quarry hounds in England and dogs on premises with horses affected by influenza in Australia in 2007 [40–44]. Interspecies transmission of equine influenza virus to dogs upon close contact with experimentally infected horses was demonstrated [45]. To date, there is no documented evidence on the transmission of equine influenza virus from dogs to horses [46].

During 2004–2006 swine influenza surveillance in central China, two equine H3N8 influenza viruses were isolated from pigs [47]. Pigs have both sialic acid (SA) a2-3 galactose and a2-6 galactose containing receptors on cell surfaces. However, in vivo infection experiments on mini-pigs demonstrated that equine influenza virus failed to induce pyrexia, appreciable histopathological lesions or virus shedding [1]. The H3 HA has broad pathogenic potential but analysis of the HA genes of influenza A viruses suggests that the equine and canine H3 have evolved separately to the H3 of avian, human and swine viruses [48].

It is generally accepted that there is a correlation between receptor binding characteristics and host specificity of equine influenza viruses. For influenza viruses to enter host cells, the HA glycoprotein must bind to sialic acid receptors on the cell surface. Viruses isolated from wild aquatic birds bind strongly to SA in a 2,3-linkage (SA 2,3). The same linkage is recognised by equine influenza virus and is the predominant linkage found on cells lining the equine upper respiratory tract. In contrast, human-adapted influenza viruses recognise and bind SA 2,6 receptors, and these are the receptors that predominate in the human respiratory tract [37]. Virus shedding and seroconversions were recorded in human volunteers inoculated with equine influenza virus [49] but although the potential for such transmission is demonstrable, there is no evidence that horses are reservoirs of virus for humans.

It is equally possible that a new influenza sub-type could emerge in horses from the avian reservoir. Although it did not replace the current equine H3N8 virus that has been circulating in horses for many years [39], cross-species transmission of avian H3N8 influenza virus into horses occurred in Jilin Province in China during 1989. The genetic analysis of the strain responsible of this outbreak (A/equine 2/Jilin 89) indicated was more closely related to avian influenza viruses than to other equine H3N8 influenza viruses [50, 51]. This strain (A/equine 2/Jilin 89) did not appear to persist in the horse population after 1990 or to spread beyond China to other countries. This transient re-emergence of the H3N8 subtype rather than any other may reflect the fact that this sub-type is commonly isolated from the avian reservoir [52]. More recently, avian H5N1 has been associated with respiratory disease in donkeys in Egypt [2]. This detection described a new subtype of highly contagious avian influenza virus as an equine infectious agent, and raises questions about the role of donkey in the spread of H5N1 virus to birds, humans and other mammals including equines.

2.3. Spread and transmission of equine influenza viruses

Influenza is primarily a seasonal disease usually occurring in epidemic form, often rampant in waves, followed by periods of relative calm. EIV is highly contagious and is primarily spread by the respiratory route through direct contact between infectious and susceptible horses in close proximity. In unvaccinated, susceptible horses, the short incubation period and persistent coughing which releases large amounts of virus into the environment contribute to the rapid spread of the infection. Personnel and fomites also contribute to virus spread. In the absence of release of horses from the quarantine station, it was concluded that the virus escaped on the person, clothing or equipment of a groom, veterinarian, farrier or someone else who had contact with the infected horses and left the station without implementing adequate biosecurity measures. The contaminated vehicles were implicated in the spread of the virus [20, 53]. Severe outbreaks of equine influenza occur in unimmunized populations of horses or when a new strain infects a vaccinated population. In a susceptible group of horses, morbidity can be as high as 100%. Horses stabled under intensive conditions are at risk from a build-up of infective virus in the common airspace. The global distribution of the EIV is associated with increased movement of horses participating in competitions or for breeding or sale. In the first outbreak of equine influenza in Australia in 2007, the initial spread of the virus in the general horse population, then spread to the Thoroughbred population, it was estimated that over 75,000 horses had been infected. In the Japanese outbreak, in the same year, the reverse situation pertained, the initial outbreaks were in racehorses and the virus then spread to the non-Thoroughbred population. In the second confirmed outbreak of respiratory disease in Algeria in 2011 since 1972, the disease occurred in a variety of locations and stud farms among Thoroughbred and non-Thoroughbred horse populations. Around 900 horses have been affected during this outbreak which led to race cancellation in the whole country for 2 months [15]. During the outbreak in Uruguay in 2012, which affected over 2000 horses, race meetings were cancelled for several weeks and movement of horses out of the country was prohibited. Equine influenza outbreaks also resulted in the cancellation of equestrian events in Brazil [27].

2.4. Mortality to EIV

Mortality is very rarely associated with equine influenza but a small number of fatalities have been reported in young foals from non-vaccinated mares; thus, inadequate passive transfer of antibodies, due to poor-quality colostrum or inadequate intake, is likely to be a major factor. All mares should be vaccinated adequately to ensure that there are sufficient maternally derived antibodies in colostrum [54, 55]. Deaths of those foals as a result of acutely viral pneumonia, and in affected donkeys and horses that are not adequately rested. In northeastern China in 1989, a mortality rate of up to 20% in some herds was associated with a large outbreak of equine influenza. More than 40 horses died during an outbreak affecting over 74,000 horses in Mongolia in 2011 [32]. Disconcertingly, several foal deaths were also reported during EI outbreaks in France during 2012 [56].

2.5. Factors influencing transmission

Although equine influenza virus spread is frequently explosive in naïve populations, the majority of outbreaks in endemic populations are contained with limited spread between premises. Outbreaks are often associated with the introduction of new horses to premises [17], and seronegative horses are frequently the index cases [57]. Although the index cases may not be the source of the virus, they act to amplify the virus and serve as a source of infection to other horses in the cohort. The severity of the disease depends on the immune status of the horse (naive, partially immunized or immunosuppressive), on the infecting viral dose, virulence of the virus strain and to the inoculation route. However, antigenic variants can give rise to large-scale disease epidemics such as occurred in 1979–1981 in Europe and in North America [58, 59]. Mismatch between vaccine and infecting strains requires higher levels of antibodies to prevent infection and significantly increases the risk of an outbreak at the population level [60, 61]. Introduction of subclinical affected vaccinated horses in a susceptible population is also a major contributing factor to influenza outbreaks, in South Africa in 1986, India in 1987, Europe in 1989, Croatia in 2004, Italy in 2005 and also suspected in Australia in 2007. In general, young horses, horses with low serum antibody titres and those that are highly mobile and mix with large groups of horses are considered most at risk [15, 62]. However, in the 2003 outbreak in Newmarket, 2-year-old horses were less susceptible than older horses despite having accounted for any differences in antibody levels [63]. Finally, a few studies demonstrated that the sex as a risk factor for influenza infection.

2.6. Survival and persistence of EIV

The equine influenza virus has a lipid envelope and does not survive for long outside the horse. It is fragile and easily inactivated by exposure to ultraviolet light for 30 min, by heating at 50°C for 30 min, by ether and by acid (pH 3). Exposure to sunlight for 15 min at 15°C also inactivates the virus. The virus will not survive long in the environment in conditions of high humidity [64].

The virus can however survive on skin, fabrics and the surfaces of contaminated equipment for some time. The periods of survival are shorter in conditions of higher humidity. Studies have also shown that the virus may be transferred from stainless steel surfaces to hands and from paper tissues to hands.

Equine influenza is a self-limiting disease and the virus does not persist in recovered horses. It is thought that influenza persists in endemic populations by low-grade circulation with occasional small outbreaks [65]. In countries where equine influenza appears not to be endemic and quarantine measures are implemented, there is no evidence of long-term persistence following sporadic incursions. In Australia in 2007, the disease was eradicated within 4 months following the implementation of an extensive control programme [66].

No information is available about the persistence of EI virus in horse carcases. Virus could be expected to be present in the carcases of animals that die during the viraemic phase of infection.

3. Conclusion

Equine influenza A H3N8 viruses continue to cause serious diseases in horses despite control measures, including quarantine and vaccination, and the international spread of the virus occurs during exchanges and participation horses in competitions. Moreover, monitoring antigenic drift and emergence of new strains that allow the production of effective vaccines is critical. Finally, the vaccination of horses by modern and effective vaccines will considered to be a new weapon to control this disease.

Author details

Farouk Laabassi

Address all correspondence to: flaabassi@yahoo.fr

ESPA Laboratory, Veterinary Department, University of Batna-1, Batna, Algeria

References

[1] Cullinane A, Newton JR. Equine influenza—a global perspective. Veterinary Microbiology. 2013; 167(1–2): 205–214.

[2] Abdelmoneim AS, Abdel-ghany AE, Shany ASS. Isolation and characterisation of highly pathogenic avian influenza subtype H5N1 from donkeys. Journal of Biomedical Science. 2010; 17(1): 25.

[3] Sovinova O, Tumova B, Pouska F. Isolation of a virus causing respiratory disease in horses. Acta Virologica. 1958; 2: 52–61.

[4] Webster RG. Are equine1 influenza viruses still present in horses? Equine Vetinary Journal. 1993; 25: 537–538.

[5] Singh G. Characterization of A/eq-1 virus isolated during the equine influenza epidemic in India. Acta Virologica. 1994; 38: 25–26.

[6] Mumford J, Wood J. Conference report on WHO/OIE meeting: consultation a newly strains of equine influenza. Vaccine. 1993; 11: 1172–1175.

[7] Madic J, Martinovic S, Naglilc T, Hajsig D, Cvetnic S. Serological evidence for the presence of A/equine-I influenza virus in unvaccinated horses in Croatia. Veterinary Record. 1996; 138: 68.

[8] Wadell GH, Teigland MB, Sigel MM. A new influenza virus associated with equine respiratory disease. Journal of American Veterinary Medicine Association. 1963; 143: 587–590.

[9] Newton JR, Daly JM, Spencer L, Mumford JA. Description of the outbreak of equine influenza (H3N8) in the United Kingdom in 2003, during which recently vaccinated horses in Newmarket developed respiratory disease. Veterinary Record. 2006; 158: 185–192.

[10] Gildea S, Quinlivan M, Arkins S, Cullinane A. The molecular epidemiology of Equine influenza in Ireland from 2007–2010 and its international significance. Equine Veterinary Journal. 2012; 44: 387–392.

[11] Damiani AM, Scicluna MT, Ciabatti I, Cardeti G, Sala M, Vulcano G, Cordioli P, Martella V, Amaddeo D, Autorino GL. Genetic characterization of equine influenza viruses isolated in Italy between 1999 and 2005. Virus Research. 2008; 131: 100–105.

[12] Ito M, Nagai M, Hayakawa Y, Komae H, Murakami N, Yotsuya S, Asakura S, Sakoda Y, Kida H. Genetic Analyses of an H3N8 influenza virus isolate, causative strain of the outbreak of equine influenza at the Kanazawa Racecourse in Japan in 2007. Journal of Veterinary Medicine Science. 2008; 70: 899–906.

[13] Rozek W, Purzycka M, Polak MP, Gradzki Z, Zmudzinski JF. Genetic typing of equine influenza virus isolated in Poland in 2005 and 2006. Virus Research. 2009; 145: 121–126.

[14] Garner MG, Cowled B, East IJ, Moloney BJ, Kung NY. Evaluating the effectiveness of early vaccination in the control and eradication of equine influenza a modelling approach. Preventive Veterinary Medicine. 2011; 99: 15–27.

[15] Laabassi F, Lecouturier F, Amelot G, Gaudaire D, Mamache B, Laugier C, Legrand L, Zientara S, Hans A. Epidemiology and genetic characterization of H3N8 equine influenza virus responsible for clinical disease in Algeria in 2011. Transboundary and Emerging Diseases. 2015; 62(6): 623–631.

[16] Daly JM, Lai AC, Binns MM, Chambers TM, Barrandeguy M, Mumford JA. Antigenic and genetic evolution of equine H3N8 influenza A viruses. Journal of General Virology. 1996; 77: 661–671.

[17] Bryant NA, Rash AS, Russell CA, Ross J, Cooke A, Bowman S, Macrae S, Lewis NS, Paillot R, Zanoni R, Meier H, Griffiths LA, Daly JM, Tiwari A, Chambers TM, Newton JR, Elton DM. Antigenic and genetic variations in European and North American equine influenza virus strains (H3N8) isolated from 2006 to 2007. Veterinary Microbiology. 2009; 138: 41–52.

[18] Lai ACK, Chambers TM, Holland JRE, Morley PS, Haines DM, Towensend HG, Barrandeguy M. Diverged evolution of recent equine-2 influenza (H3N8) viruses in the Western Hemisphere. Archives of Virology. 2001; 146: 1063–1074.

[19] Muller I, Pinto E, Santibanez MC, Celedon MO, Valenzuela PD. Isolation and characterization of the equine influenza virus causing the 2006 outbreak in Chile. Veterinary Microbiology. 2009; 137: 172–177.

[20] King E, Macdonald D. Report of the Board of Inquiry appointed by the Board of the National Horseracing Authority to conduct enquiry into the causes of the equine influenza which started in the Western Cape in early December 2003 and spread to the Eastern Cape and Gauteng. Australian Equine Veterinary. 2004; 23:139–142.

[21] Jeggo MH, Hammond JM, Kirkland PD. The initial laboratory diagnosis of equine influenza in Australia in 2007. Microbiology Australia. 2008; 29: 80–82.

[22] Yamanaka T, Niwa H, Tsujimura K, Kondo T, Matsumura T. Epidemic of equine influenza among vaccinated racehorses in Japan in 2007. Journal of Veterinary Medicine Science. 2008; 70: 623–625.

[23] Bryant NA, Rash AS, Woodward AL, Medcalf E, Helwegen M, Wohlfender F, Cruz F, Herrmann C, Borchers K, Tiwari A, Chambers TM, Newton JR, Mumford JA, Elton DM. Isolation and characterisation of equine influenza viruses (H3N8) from Europe and North America from 2008 to 2009. Veterinary Microbiology. 2011; 147: 19–27.

[24] Watson J, Halpin K, Selleck P, Axell A, Bruce K, Hansson E, Hammond J, Daniels P, Jeggo M. Isolation and characterisation of an H3N8 Equine influenza virus in Australia, 2007. Australian Veterinary Journal. 2011; 89(Suppl. 1): 35–37.

[25] Legrand LJ, Pitel PHY, Marcillaud-Pitel CJ, Cullinane AA, Courouce AM, Fortier GD, Freymuth FL, Pronost SL. Surveillance of equine influenza viruses through the RESPE

network in France from November 2005 to October 2010. Equine Veterinary Journal. 2013; 45: 776–783.

[26]   Back H, Treiberg Berndtsson L, Gröndahl G, Ståhl K, Pringle J, Zohari S. The first reported Florida clade 1 virus in the Nordic countries, isolated from a Swedish outbreak of equine influenza in 2011. Veterinary Microbiology. 2016; 184: 1–6.

[27]   Alves Beuttemmüller E, Woodward A, Rash A, Ferraz LES, Alfieri AF, Alfieri AC, Elton D. Characterisation of the epidemic strain of H3N8 equine influenza virus responsible for outbreaks in South America in 2012. Virology Journal. 2016; 13: 45.

[28]   Qi T, Guo W, Huang WQ, Li HM, Zhao LP, Dai LL, He N, Hao XF, Xiang WH. Isolation and genetic characterization of H3N8 equine influenza virus from donkeys in China. Veterinary Microbiology. 2010; 144: 455–460.

[29]   Virmani N, Bera BC, Singh BK, Shanmugasundaram K, Gulati BR, Barua S, Vaid RK, Gupta AK, Singh RK. Equine influenza outbreak in India (2008–2009): virus isolation, sero-epidemiology and phylogenetic analysis of HA gene. Veterinary Microbiology. 2010; 143: 224–237.

[30]   Wei G, Xue-Feng L, Yan Y, Ying-Yuan W, Ling-Li D, Li-Ping Z, Wen-Hua X, Jian-Hua Z. Equine influenza viruses isolated during outbreaks in China in 2007 and 2008. Veterinary Record. 2010; 167: 382–383.

[31]   Bountouri M, Fragkiadaki E, Ntafis V, Kanellos T, Xylouri E. Phylogenetic and molecular characterization of Equine H3N8 influenza viruses from Greece (2003 and 2007): evidence for reassortment between evolutionary lineages. Virology Journal. 2011; 8: 350.

[32]   Yondon M, Heil GL, Burks JP, Zayat B, Waltzek TB, Jamiyan BO, McKenzie PP, Krueger WS, Friary JA, Gray JC. Isolation and characterization of H3N8 Equine influenza A virus associated with the 2011 epizootic in Mongolia. Influenza and Other Respiratory Viruses. 2013; 7: 659–665.

[33]   Zientara S. Molecular epidemiology: the example of equine influenza. Epidémiologie et santé animale. 2001; 39: 69–74.

[34]   Francis T, Salk JE, Pearson HE, Brown PN. Protective effect of vaccination against induced influenza A. Journal of Clinical Investigation. 1945; 24: 536–546.

[35]   Cullinane A, Elton D, Mumford J. Equine influenza – surveillance and control. Influenza and Other Respiratory Viruses. 2010; 4: 339–344.

[36]   Hannant D, Mumford JA. Equine influenza. In: Studdert M, editor. Virus Infections of Equines. Amsterdam: Elsevier Science; 1996. p. 285–293.

[37]   Daly JM, MacRae S, Newton JR, Wattrang E, Elton DM. Equine influenza: a review of an unpredictable virus. The Veterinary Journal. 2011; 189: 7–14.

[38] Laabassi F, Mamache B. Equine influenza virus: epidemiology, diagnosis and vaccination. Revue de Médecine Vétérinaire. 2014 ; 165(1–2): 31–43.

[39] Gorman OT, Bean WJ, Kawaoka Y, Donatelli I, Guo Y, Webster RG. Evolution of influenza A virus nucleoprotein genes: implications for the origins of H1N1 human and classical swine viruses. Journal of Virology. 1991; 65: 3704–3714.

[40] Crawford PC, Dubovi EJ, Castleman WL, Stephenson I, Gibbs EP, Chen L, Smith C, Hill RC, Ferro P, Pompey J, Bright RA, Medina MJ, Johnson CM, Olsen CW, Cox NJ, Klimov AI, Katz JM, Donis RO. Transmission of equine influenza virus to dogs. Science. 2005; 310: 482–485.

[41] Smith DJ, Lapedes AS, de Jong JC, Bestebroer TM, Rimmelzwaan GF, Osterhaus ADME, Fouchier RAM. Mapping the antigenic and genetic evolution of influenza virus. Science. 2004; 305: 371–376.

[42] Newton R, Cooke A, Elton D, Bryant N, Rash A, Bowman S, Blunden T, Miller J, Hammond TA, Camm I, Day M. Canine influenza virus: cross-species transmission from horses. Veterinary Record. 2007; 161: 142–143.

[43] Daly JM, Blunden AS, Macrae S, Miller J, Bowman SJ, Kolodziejek J, Nowotny N, Smith KC. Transmission of equine influenza virus to English foxhounds. Emerging Infectious Diseases. 2008; 14: 461–464.

[44] Kirkland PD, Finlaison DS, Crispe E, Hunt AC. Influenza virus transmission from horses to dogs, Australia. Emerging Infectious Diseases. 2010; 16: 699–702.

[45] Yamanaka T, Nemoto M, Tsujimura K, Kondo T, Matsumura T. Interspecies transmission of equine influenza virus (H3N8) to dogs by close contact with experimentally infected horses. Veterinary Microbiology. 2009; 139: 351–355.

[46] Yamanaka T, Nemoto M, Bannai H, Tsujimura K, Kondo T, Matsumura T, Muranaka M, Ueno T, Kinoshita Y, Niwa H, Hidari KI, Suzuki T. No evidence of horizontal infection in horses kept in close contact with dogs experimentally infected with canine influenza A virus (H3N8). Acta Veterinaria Scandinavica. 2012; 54: 25.

[47] Tu J, Zhou H, Jiang T, Li C, Zhang A, Guo X, Zou W, Chen H, Jin M. Isolation and molecular characterization of equine H3N8 influenza viruses from pigs in China. Archives of Virology. 2009; 154: 887–890.

[48] Shi W, Lei F, Zhu C, Sievers F, Higgins DG. A complete analysis of HA and NA genes of influenza A viruses. PLoS ONE. 2010; 5: e14454.

[49] Kasel JA, Couch RB. Experimental infection in man and horses with influenza A viruses. The Bulletin of the World Health Organization. 1969; 41: 447–452.

[50] Webster RG, Guo YJ. New influenza virus in horses. Nature. 1991; 351: 527.

[51] Guo Y, Wang M, Kawaoka Y, Gorman O, Ito T, Saito T, Webster RG. Characterization of a new avian-like influenza A virus from horses in China. Virology. 1992; 188: 245–255.

[52] Sharp GB, Kawaoka Y, Jones DJ, Bean WJ, Pryor SP, Hinshaw V, Webster RG. Coinfection of wild ducks by influenza A viruses: distribution patterns and biological significance. Journal of Virology. 1997; 71: 6128–6135.

[53] Guthrie AJ, Stevens KB, Bosman PP. The circumstances surrounding the outbreak and spread of equine influenza in South Africa. Revue Scientifique Technique. 1999; 18: 179–185.

[54] Patterson-Kane JC, Carrick JB, Axon JE, Wilkie I, Begg AP. The pathology of bronchointerstitial pneumonia in young foals associated with the first outbreak of equine influenza in Australia. Equine Veterinary Journal. 2008; 40: 199–203.

[55] Slater J, Borchers K, Chambers T, Cullinane A, Duggan V, Elton D, Legrand L, Paillot R, Fortier G. Report of the International Equine Influenza Roundtable Expert Meeting at Le Touquet, Normandy, February 2013. Equine Veterinary Journal. 2014; 46: 645–650.

[56] Legrand L, Fougerolles S, Hans A, Le Net JL, Gaudaire D, Foucher N, Roussel C, Pronost S, Tapprest J. Description of an episode of equine influenza in a Normandy breeding with foals fatalities. In: Proceedings of Annual Days of French Equine Veterinary Association (AVEF); 11–13 December 2013, Deauville; 2013. p. 255–256.

[57] Wood JLN. A review of the history and epidemiology and a description of recent outbreak (MSc Dissertation). London: University of London; 1991.

[58] Burrows R, Goodridge D, Denyer M, Hutchings G, Frank CJ. Equine influenza infections in Great Britain, 1979. Veterinary Record. 1982; 110: 494–497.

[59] Hinshaw VS, Naeve CW, Webster RG, Douglas A, Skehel JJ, Bryans J. Analysis of antigenic variation in equine 2 influenza A viruses. The Bulletin of the World Health Organization. 1983; 61: 153–158.

[60] Newton JR, Verheyen K, Wood JL, Yates PJ, Mumford JA. Equine influenza in the United Kingdom in 1998. Veterinary Record. 1999; 145: 449–452.

[61] Park AW, Wood JL, Daly JM, Newton JR, Glass K, Henley W, Mumford JA, Grenfell BT. The effects of strain heterology on the epidemiology of equine influenza in a vaccinated population. Proceedings of the Biological Sciences. 2004; 271: 1547–1555.

[62] Morley PS, Townsend HG, Bogdan JR, Haines DM. Risk factors for disease associated with influenza virus infections during three epidemics in horses. Journal of the American Veterinary Medicine Association. 2000; 216: 545–550.

[63] Barquero N, Daly JM, Newton JR. Risk factors for influenza infection in vaccinated racehorses: lessons from an outbreak in Newmarket, UK in 2003. Vaccine. 2007; 25: 7520–7529.

[64] Yadav MP, Uppal PK, Mumford JA. Physico-chemical and biological characterization of A/Equi-2 virus isolated from 1987 equine influenza epidemic in India. International Journal of Animal Science. 1993; 8: 93–98.

[65] Glass K, Wood JL, Mumford JA, Jesset D, Grenfell BT. Modelling equine influenza 1: a stochastic model of within-yard epidemics. Epidemiology & Infection. 2002; 128: 491–502.

[66] Garner MG, Cowled B, East IJ, Moloney BJ, Kung NY. Evaluating the effectiveness of early vaccination in the control and eradication of equine influenza—a modelling approach. Preventive Veterinary Medicine. 2011; 99: 15–27.

Chapter 3

Epidemiology and Emergence of Schmallenberg Virus Part 1: Origin, Transmission and Differential Diagnosis

Fernando Esteves, João Rodrigo Mesquita,
Cármen Nóbrega, Carla Santos, António Monteiro,
Rita Cruz, Helena Vala and Ana Cláudia Coelho

Additional information is available at the end of the chapter

http://dx.doi.org/10.5772/64741

Abstract

Schmallenberg virus (SBV) is a novel *Orthobunyavirus* causing mild clinical signs in cows and malformations in aborted and neonatal ruminants in Europe. SBV belongs to the family Bunyaviridae and is transmitted by biting midges. This new virus was identified for the first time in the blood samples of cows in the city of Schmallenberg in North-Rhine-Westphalia in November 2011. Since then the virus spread to several European countries. Here we describe the origin and emergence, as well as the transmission and the differential diagnosis of this virus, now known to be a serious threat to Veterinary Public Health.

Keywords: Schmallenberg virus, emerging infections, epidemiology

1. Introduction

1.1. The origin of Schmallenberg virus

In 2011, an unidentified disease in cattle was reported in Germany and the Netherlands [1]. Hyperthermia and drop in milk production were reported in adult dairy cows in north-west Germany and the Netherlands, and in some cases, transient diarrhoea was also recorded in the Netherlands [2]. Farmers and veterinarians in North Rhine-Westphalia, Germany, and in the Netherlands reported an unidentified disease in dairy cattle with a short period of clear clinical signs to the animal health services, local diagnostic laboratories and national research institutes

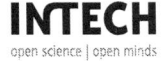

[1]. All classical endemic and emerging viruses, such as pestiviruses, bovine herpesvirus type-1 (BHV-1), foot-and-mouth disease (FMD) virus, bluetongue virus (BTV), epizootic haemorrhagic disease (EHD) virus, Rift Valley fever (RVF) virus and bovine ephemeral fever (BEF) virus, could be excluded as the causative agent [1].

The first identification of this new virus succeeded in samples of cattle housed next to a small town in Germany with 25,000 inhabitants, called Schmallenberg, in North Rhine-Westphalia (**Figure 1**).

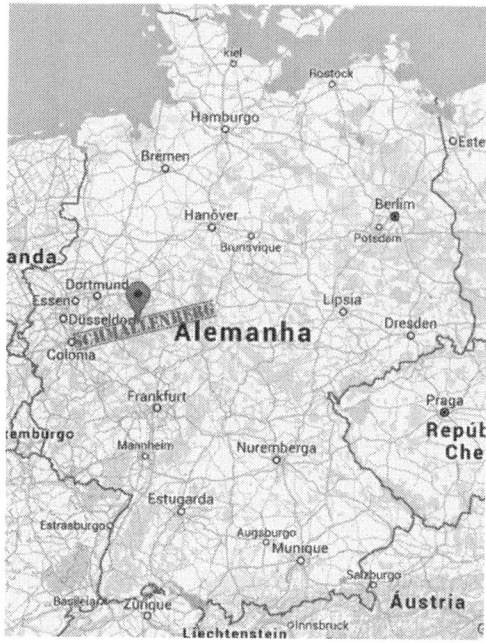

Figure 1. Location of Schmallenberg city, North Rhine-Westphalia, Germany.

At that time and following elimination of the usual causes of such clinical signs in cattle, blood samples from three bovine were subjected to the new technology of deep sequencing known as metagenomic analysis, which allows the sequencing of all nucleic acids present in a sample [3]. Metagenomics is the application of modern genomics techniques to the study of communities of microbial organisms directly in their natural environments, bypassing the need for isolation and lab cultivation of individual species [4]. As is typical with this approach, a large amount of host genomic and known bacterial sequences were identified, the latter most likely as a consequence of prolonged sample storage. However, present within the samples were genetic sequences from a novel *Bunyavirus* which had the highest homology to viruses of the Simbu serogroup virus [3]. This novel virus was named as Schmallenberg virus (SBV), characterized by a syndrome in ruminants referred to the arthrogryposis–hydranencephaly syndrome (AHS), resulting in abortions, stillbirths and congenital defects in newborn ruminants after infection during pregnancy [5].

1.2. Structure and taxonomy

SBV is now known to belong to the genus *Orthobunyavirus* and the Bunyaviridae family, as confirmed from electron microscopy [1, 3, 6]. Most viruses of this genus have not yet been well characterized [3]. SBV is also a member of Simbu serogroup, one of the largest of the 18 serogroups which constitute the genus [3]. Simbu serogroup includes the virus Shamonda, Akabane and Aino; however, the most related to SBV are virus Sathuperi and Douglas [6]. Its reorganization capability has also been suggested [1], especially when taken into account that many strains of *Orthobunyavirus* suffered re-assortment [3, 7].

SBV is typical of the Bunyaviridae, characterized by a tripartite negative-sense RNA genome that encodes four structural and two non-structural proteins [8]. The SBV is an enveloped virus with a surface of glycoproteins [6]. The diameter of these viruses is approximately 100 nm. Their genetic structure comprises of three segments of single-stranded negative-sense RNA: large (L) with 6865 nucleotides, medium (M) with 4415 nucleotides and small (S) with 830 nucleotides (**Figure 2**) [1, 3].

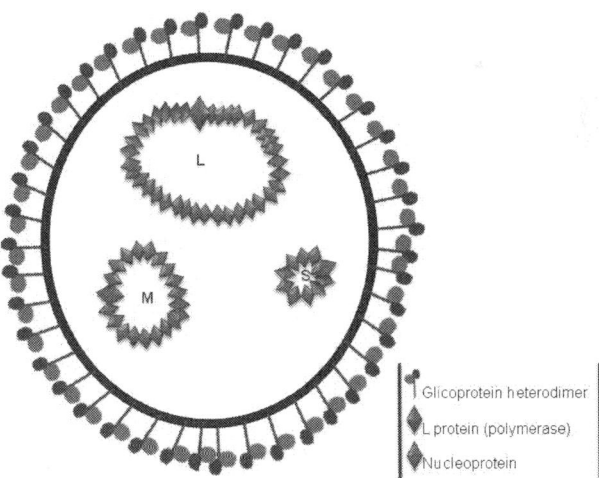

Figure 2. Diagram illustrating a particle of Schmallenberg virus with glycoproteins (Gn and Gc) and the three segments of RNA (small (S), medium (M) and large (L) in a circular form in association with nucleoprotein and the 'L' polymerase protein (adapted from Tarlinton et al. [3]).

The large (L) segment encodes the viral RNA-dependent RNA-polymerase or L protein, the medium (M) segment encodes the virion glycoproteins Gn and Gc, and the small (S) segment encodes the nucleoprotein (N). Non-structural proteins are encoded by some viruses on the M (NSm protein) and by some on the S (NSs protein) segment [8].

The full genome sequence of the first described SBV is provided under the Genbank accession number HE649912 and has a length of 6864 base pairs [1].

1.3. The emergence of Schmallenberg virus

From November 2011 to date, the disease spread rapidly and widely throughout Europe. Since 2011 cases have been reported: Belgium (December 2011), the UK and France (January 2012), Luxembourg and Italy (February 2012), Spain (March 2012), Denmark (June 2012), Switzerland and Sweden (July 2012), Austria and Finland (September 2012), Ireland and Poland (October 2012), Norway (November 2012), Czech Republic (December 2012), Estonia, Slovenia, Hungary and Croatia (January 2013), Latvia (April 2013), Greece (March 2013), Russia (May 2013), Serbia (June 2013) and Romania (July 2013) [9]. There are also reports of cases outside Europe [10]. Recently a new study shows the circulation of the virus in Portugal [11] (**Figure 3**).

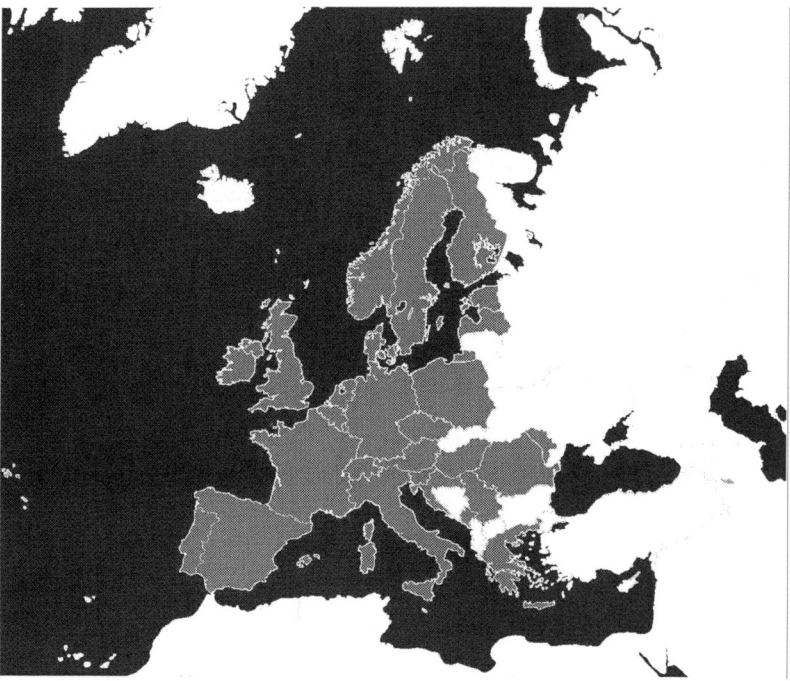

Figure 3. Distribution of the disease caused by SBV in Europe.

In the future, new outbreaks are expected depending on many conditions like the vector transmission [9].

1.4. Disease transmission

As viruses belonging to the genus *Orthobunyavirus* (e.g. Akabane virus) are widespread in Africa and Asia, and biting midges (*Culicoides* spp.) and mosquitoes are responsible for transmitting these viruses [12], it was assumed that an array of European Culicoides might be responsible for transmitting SBV within Europe.

Rasmussen et al. [13] demonstrated the presence of SBV RNA in *Culicoides obsoletus* group midges caught in Denmark during October 2011. The low C_t values (i.e. high SBV RNA levels) and the absence of ruminant β-actin mRNA in these samples strongly suggest that SBV replicates in these midges, and hence that the *C. obsoletus* group midges are natural vectors for this virus [12]. Field studies have shown the presence of SBV RNA in *Culicoides* species in several affected countries [13, 14], and a vector-competence study demonstrated replication and dissemination of SBV in laboratory Culicoides strains. Midges including *Culicoides scoticus*, *C. chiopterus* and *C. obsoletus* sensu stricto were collected in the field and tested positive for SBV in Belgium [14]. SBV-positive *Culicoides dewulfi* and *C. obsoletus* were also detected in Belgium and Denmark [13].

The transmission by a wide range of *Culicoides* spp. may explain the rapid spread of SBV.

Viruses more closely related to SBV are not considered zoonoses; hence, most authorities have concluded that the probability of SBV infecting humans is minimal [3]. Because SBV emerged recently, transmission from animals to human cannot yet be completely excluded. A seroprevalence study by Ducomble et al. [15] conducted among exposed shepherds in the area of Germany most affected by SBV showed no evidence of transmission to humans. However, further studies on whether SBV poses a risk to humans are vital [15].

1.5. Schmallenberg virus impact on ruminant health

SBV has the ability to infect exclusively ruminant species [9]. Within the domestic ruminants, the most affected are cattle, followed by sheep and goats [16]. Horizontal transmission occurs through various *Culicoides* biting midges, and subsequent transplacental transmission causes teratogenic effects. Despite infection being mostly asymptomatic, foetal Schmallenberg virus infection in naïve ewes and goats can result in stillborn offspring, showing a congenital arthrogryposis-hydranencephaly syndrome. The economic impact of infection depends on the number of malformed lambs but is generally limited [9]. It was shown that SBV infection in meat sheep herds caused increased rates of abortion, malformations, dystocia, lamb mortality and reduced fertility rate [16]. A study conducted by Wüthrich et al. [17] revealed that the average calculated loss after SBV infection for a standardized farm was EUR 1338, which can be considered low at the national level, but the losses were subject to great fluctuations between farms, so individual farms could have very high losses (EUR 8333). The overall prevalence of infected animals within a herd is an important factor [17], and the economic impact of the infection depends on several aspects, such as, the number of malformed lambs, days where milk production is lower and stage of pregnancy on which the infection occurred [9, 17]. However, the emergence of SVB has a financial impact on international trade in live sheep and goats, for example, with some countries (USA, Mexico and Japan), to place restrictions on the import of embryos and semen of Europe [9]. In conclusion, the impact of SBV on animal population and the associated economic losses are still much discussed, though surveillance activities (syndromic surveillance, abortion surveillance, sentinel herd and Culicoides surveillance) and databases as well as cross-sectional epidemiological studies on disease outbreaks are essential to analyse the real impact of these and define action steps [10, 18].

2. Differential diagnosis of SBV

The clinical symptoms of acute SBV infection are unspecific and vary among animal populations. Thus, possible causes of high fever, diarrhoea, decrease in milk production, increased incidence of abortion and congenital malformations should be taken into account in the establishment of the differential diagnosis and consequently in obtaining definitive diagnosis. In contrary to cattle, clinical signs reported in adult small ruminants may be present only during the viraemic phase, but in most cases the infection is mostly asymptomatic [9].

Malformation in newborn or stillborn lambs and clinical signs correlate with the stage of development at which the foetus was infected but these are also not specific of SBV infection. Foetal Schmallenberg virus infection in naïve ewes and goats can result in stillborn offspring, showing a congenital arthrogryposis-hydranencephaly syndrome [9]; however, other congenital malformations may be present such as hydrocephaly, brachygnathia inferior, ankylosis, torticollis and scoliosis.

The lack of specificity of the observed clinical signs in infected adults, stillborn foetuses and malformed neonates means that a definitive diagnosis of SBV infection can only be made accurately based on clinical evaluation and specific laboratory examinations [9].

Although several differential diagnosis for abortion and congenital abnormalities have been suggested to include several factors such as genetic (spider lamb syndrome), teratogenic chemicals or toxins (*Veratrum californicum*, *Lupinus* spp., pregnancy toxaemia, lead poisoning) nutritional conditions such as vitamin (vitamin A, vitamin B1) or mineral deficiencies (hypocalcaemia, hypomagnesaemia, copper) and infectious agents [19], in this section we are going to emphasize infectious causes of this condition. In general, a sudden onset of clustered cases of abortion, premature and at term, live or stillborn foetuses with arthrogryposis and hydranencephaly suggests a teratogenic virus as possible cause.

The main infectious diseases to consider include:

• **Bluetongue disease**

Bluetongue is an arthropod-borne disease affecting wild and domestic ruminants although clinical disease is present mostly in sheep; cattle and goats hosts [20, 21]. The disease occurs worldwide and is caused by bluetongue virus (BTV), which belongs to the genus *Orbivirus* within the family Reoviridae [20].

BTV infection of livestock is distinctly seasonal (late summer and fall) in the temperate region once is transmitted biologically by certain species of Culicoides midges that consequently show maximum activity in high temperature and high humidity [21–23], and these conditions can influence the activity of the vector as well as the viability of the virus. Some authors propose that the global climate changes as well as geography and altitude affect the activity of the vector and are responsible for sudden outbreaks worldwide [21, 23, 24].

The types of characteristic lesions of BTV in affected sheep include: haemorrhage and erosion/ ulcers on mucous membrane of the oral cavity and upper gastrointestinal tract, necrotic lesions on the lips, dental footpad and tongue as well as oedema [20], necrosis of skeletal and cardiac muscle, coronitis, subintimal haemorrhage in the pulmonary artery; oedema of the lungs, ventral subcutis and fascia of the muscles of the neck and abdominal wall; and pericardial, pleural and abdominal effusions [25].

Other unspecific signs include drop in milk production, loss of body weight, fever, depression, excessive salivation, serous to bloody nasal discharge, facial oedema, hyperaemia, lameness and death [20, 26]. In goats, the infection demonstrated an acute drop in milk production, oedema of the lips and head, nasal discharge and erythema of the skin and udder [20]; however, in goats and cattle infection may be unapparent [20]. Newborn lambs may reveal porencephaly and cerebral necrosis; however, this type of lesions is more frequent after vaccination using an attenuated virus. The severities of clinical signs seem to vary with the species, breed, age, immune status and the serotype/strain of the infecting virus and with certain rather ill-defined interactions with the environment. Bluetongue typically occurs when susceptible animal species are introduced into areas with circulating virulent BTV strains, or when virulent BTV strains extend their range to previously unexposed populations of ruminants [24, 27].

The outcome of BTV infection of foetal ruminants is age-dependent and transplacental infection [28], which may result in either stillbirths, abortions or the birth of non-viable lambs with severe lesions of the central nervous system [20, 25]. In cattle, most infections are unapparent [20, 21]; however, a few animals may develop clinical signs that include fever, salivation, facial oedema, lesions on lips and nostrils, ulcerations in the oral and nasal mucosa, including tongue and gingiva, and coronitis [29, 30]. In utero transmission occurs in cattle and can result in birth of viraemic calves, abortion, congenital defects such as cerebellar hypoplasia, hydranencephaly or porencephaly accompanied with behavioural abnormalities (head pressing, ataxia, inability to stand and suck well, dullness, disorientation and impaired vision)and congenital musculoskeletal deformities (agnathia, brachygnathia and arthrogry-posis) [29–31].

• **Epizootic haemorrhagic disease (EHD)**

Epizootic haemorrhagic disease virus is a member of the genus *Orbivirus*, family Reoviridae, and is closely related to bluetongue virus [32–34]. The virus is transmitted between susceptible ruminants in temperate regions by biological vectors from the genus *Culicoides* spp. [35];

therefore, this infection is most common in the late summer and autumn during peak vector population [36, 37]. Another factor that may contribute to the dissemination of this disease is the introduction of ruminants from neighbouring farms without quarantine and the presence of organic and other waste-water lagoons on the farm that can act as attraction for the mosquito [35, 37]. The main source of the virus is the blood of viraemic animals. The clinical signs of EHD in cattle are fever, anorexia, dysphagia, prostration, nasal discharge, ulcerative and necrotic lesions of the oral mucosa, hyperaemia and oedema of the conjunctival mucosae, muzzle, hyperaemia of the teats and udder, haemorrhage, dehydration and lameness [33, 35]. Abortions [38] and stillbirths have also been reported in some epidemics [39].

• **Foot and mouth disease (FMD)**

FMD is a highly contagious disease caused by an aphtovirus that belongs to the Picornaviridae family [40, 41], which affects cloven-hoofed animals, mostly cattle, swine, sheep, goats and many species of wild ungulates; however, sheep and goats can be carriers, some studies reveal that the last two species are infrequent carriers. In adult cattle, the main symptoms are characterized by a sudden decrease in milk production, fever (40–41°C), lameness, as well as severe diarrhoea and anorexia, followed by the appearance of vesicles and erosions in the mouth, teats and feet [42], and abortion in pregnant animals. Secondary infections can appear in these areas in which the more notable one is the acute painful stomatitis. Although FMDV rarely causes death in adult animals, young animals are more susceptible and may suffer from severe lesions in the myocardium [42]. Reproductive failure and abortion may also be reported [43–45].

In sheep and goats, the disease is generally mild and is important mainly because of the risk of transmission to cattle and can be difficult to distinguish from other common conditions [41, 46].The more common syndrome in this species is the appearance of a few small lesions, but with a more severe involvement of all four feet. The principal mechanism of transmission is the respiratory route [41, 47] or by ingestion through direct or indirect contact with secretions or excretions from infected animals; however, the possibility of aerogenous infection exists between cloven-hoofed species [48]. Cattle are the most susceptible, followed by sheep, whereas pigs are very resistant [47]. The period of maximum infectivity occurs during the early clinical phase of the disease when there is contact with the vesicular fluid when vesicles are discharged.

• **Bovine viral diarrhoea (BVD) and Border disease virus of sheep**

These viruses are members of the Flaviviridae family and belong to *Pestivirus* genus. BVD infects a range of domestic and wild ruminants [49]. Among the ruminant pestiviruses, there are two biotypes designated as non-cytopathic and cytopathic depending on their effect on tissue culture cells. Only the non-cytopathic, which is ubiquitous in nature, has the ability to establish persistent infection, once this type crosses the placenta invades the foetus and establishes persistent infection due to the non-recognition of the virus, at the age of infection, by the immature immune system. This condition is determinant for the spread of the virus [50,

51]. Cytopathic bovine viral diarrhoea virus (BVDV) is rare and seldom isolated unless accompanied by non-cytopathic BVDV.

Although clinical presentations depend on several factors, such as on strain of virus, species of host, immune status of host, reproductive status of host, age of host, concomitant infections and time of gestation [49], BVD virus is known to produce from subclinical infections (persistently infected animals) to a large number of diverse diseases, including reproductive disorders (decrease in conception rate and pregnancy rate, increased embryonic mortality), early embryonic death, foetal reabsorption abortion, stillbirths, central nervous system defects (microencephaly, cerebellar hypoplasia, hydranencephaly, hydrocephalus, hypomyelinogenesis, hypomyelination, cerebellar-ocular agenesis, ocular abnormalities), ocular abnormalities (microphthalmia, cataracts, retinal degeneration, optic neuritis), musculoskeletal deformities (brachygnatism), thymic aplasia, hypotrichosis, alopecia, pulmonary and renal hypoplasia [29, 50], growth retardation [29], enteritis and mucosal disease [51–53]. The most dramatic clinical symptoms are associated with the peracute form of the disease that is characterized by a sudden decrease in milk production, fever, watery and bloody diarrhoea, dehydration, tenesmus, tachypnea, tachycardia, drooping ears, anorexia, excessive lacrimation, nasal discharge, hypersalivation, petechial and ecchymotic haemorrhages of the visible mucosa, and development of ulcers of the nares, muzzle, lips and oral cavity [54] mucous membranes as well as skin lesions around the inguinal and perineal regions, the inner thighs and inside the ears [55]. Thrombocytopenia and haemorrhagic syndrome [54] may also be present in animals affected with the disease. Mucosal disease may also appear as a chronic form which persists for weeks to months and is manifested by inappetence, intermittent to chronic diarrhoea and weight loss. Cattle that have chronic mucosal disease appear unthrifty, may show lameness due to laminitis or interdigital necrosis, and may develop alopecia and hyperkeratinization. Acute or chronic mucosal disease usually occurs in cattle younger than 3 years of age [55].

The virus is transmitted by direct contact between animals and by transplacental transmission to the foetuses. The primary source of infection is the introduction of persistently infected animals into the farm [56]. Nose-to-nose contact is the most effective method of transmitting the virus. Another way of transmission is through contact with fomites such as contaminated needles, obstetric gloves or other equipment [53, 57]. Another indirect way of contact is the transmission through blood-feeding flies and artificial insemination [56].

Border disease (BD) is a congenital virus disease of sheep and goats and is caused by a pestivirus closely related to classical swine fever virus and bovine viral diarrhoea virus [58]. Ewes in acute infection are clinically normal, and viraemia is transient and difficult to detect, and the infection in goats is rare and mainly characterized by abortion. Clinical signs in sheep include barren ewes, abortions, stillbirths, birth of unviable lambs, foetal death with resorption and mummification [58–60]. Affected newborn lambs can show clonic rythmic tremors, abnormal body conformation, inability to stand, gait anomalies and abnormally hairy birthcoat so-called 'hairy-shaker' or 'fuzzy' lambs which is due to hypertrophy of primary follicles and medullation of wool fibres [61]. Nervous signs are due to a defective myelinogenesis and tend to disappear at a later age [61–63]. Some authors showed that major skeletal abnormalities are brachygnathia, prognathia and arthrogryposis [59]. Although some lambs die shortly after birth, surviving lambs, as well as apparently normal lambs, can be persistently infected with the virus and excrete it constantly for the rest of their lives. The virus is excreted with saliva, nasal discharge, urine and faeces [63]. Persistently infected animals are the major source of infection and are responsible for the vertical transmission to other susceptible flock or even cattle when mixed grazing is present [60]. The surviving lambs are persistently infected with the virus. Acute infection is usually subclinical, and sheep may also be infected following a close contact with cattle excreting the closely related BVDV [60].

• **Bovine herpesvirus type-1 and other herpesviruses**

Infectious bovine rhinotracheitis/infectious pustularvulvovaginitis (IBR/IPV) is caused by bovine herpesvirus type-1 (BHV-1) [64], and is a disease of domestic and wild cattle. BoHV-1 is a member of the genus *Varicellovirus*, which belongs to the Herpesviridae family, subfamily Alphaherpesvirinae [50, 64]. BHV-1 shares antigenic and genetic close relationships with other ruminant alphaherpesviruses [64]: BoHV-5, caprine herpesvirus-1, cervid herpesvirus-1 (red deer), cervid herpesvirus-2 (reindeer), bubaline herpesvirus-1 and elk herpesvirus-1 [65]. The virus has been associated with a wide range of clinical symptoms, including rhinotracheitis, abortion, infertility and occasionally encephalitis in calves [50, 66]. However, the clinical symptoms may be mild and localized or include severe generalized disease, leading eventually to death [67]. Infection of cattle by bovine herpesvirus type-1 (BHV-1) can lead to upper respiratory tract disorders (rhinitis, tracheitis, mucopurulent nasal discharge and conjunctivitis) [68], conjunctivitis, genital disorders (endometritis, poor conception rates, pustularvulvovaginitis, balanoposthitis) and immune suppression [65]. The main sources of infection to susceptible animals are those with a latent BHV-1 and the contact with nasal secretions, coughed-up droplets, genital secretions, semen, genital fluids and tissues of infected animals [69].

In adult goats, infection with caprineherpesvirus-1 (BHV-6) is responsible for abortion during the second half of pregnancy, stillbirth and neonatal deaths, and the infection leads to vulvovaginitis [70] or balanoposthitis [65]. In newborn kids, ulcerative and necrotic lesions [71] are distributed throughout the enteric tract, and a complex and purulent respiratory compromise and systemic disease is present [65].

• **Rift Valley fever**

Rift Valley fever (RVF) virus belongs to the *Phlebovirus* genus and Bunyaviridae family and is a vector-borne disease of sheep, cattle and goats [72]. The disease is usually present in epizootic form over large areas of a country following heavy rains and sustained flooding, and is characterized by high rates of abortion, neonatal mortality, primarily in sheep once these are more susceptible than cattle and goats [73]. Besides domestic and wild ruminants, humans can also be infected [72]. The disease is also characterized by foetal malformation accompanied by high mortality, bloody diarrhoea, haemorrhages and acute hepatic necrosis [72, 73]. The most frequent foetal abnormalities include cerebellar hypoplasia, por- or hydranencephaly and skeletal deformities such as brachygnathia and arthrogryposis [31].

Many species of mosquitoes have been identified as vectors [73, 74]. Some *Aedes* species act as reservoirs for the virus during inter-epidemic periods, and increased rainfall in dry areas leads to an explosive hatching of mosquito eggs, many of which contain the virus. The infected *Aedes* spp. feed preferentially on domestic ruminants which act as an amplifier of the virus [74]. Humans infect themselves through direct or indirect (aerosols) contact with blood, secretions or tissues of infected animals, which occurs in veterinary procedures (obstetrical manoeuvres, medical treatments), animal husbandry [75], slaughtering, consumption of raw milk and in food preparation. Another source of infection for humans and livestock is the infected blood sucking mosquitoes' vector [76].

In general, clinical signs of the disease tend to be unspecific; however, the sudden onset of numerous abortions (with rates near 100%) and high mortality among young animals along with the clinical history and the environmental factors can help in the establishment of the clinical diagnoses. In sheep, the most common symptoms are (highly susceptible) fever (40–41°C), inappetence, nasal discharge, incoordination, weakness, depression, bloody or fetid diarrhoea [76]. Newborn lambs are considered extremely susceptible, and the main symptoms are: sudden death, fever prior to death (40–42°C), weakness, depression, listless, abdominal pain, tachypnea, increased respiratory rate abdominal respiration prior to death [72].

- **Bovine ephemeral fever (BEF)**

BEF is an arthropod-borne rhabdovirus that causes a debilitant disease of cattle and water buffaloes with considerable economic impact [77–79]. Bovine ephemeral fever virus belongs to *Ephemerovirus* genus from the Rhabdoviridae family. The virus has been isolated from a range of potential insect vectors, including a large number of species of Culicoides and several species of mosquitoes such as *Aedes* spp., *Culex* spp. and *Anopheles* spp. [79]. Bovine ephemeral fever virus causes a febrile illness affecting mainly mature animals [80]. The onset of clinical signs is usually rapid: a sudden sharp drop in milk production, loss of condition fever stiffness, lameness, nasal and ocular discharges, periorbital swelling, sialorrhea, tachypnea, dyspnoea, nasal and ocular discharges, depression, cessation of rumination and constipation [77, 81, 82]. Cows in advanced pregnancy may abort [77].

- **Akabane virus**

Akabane virus is an *Orthobunyavirus* and member of the Simbu serogroup of the family Bunyaviridae. Akabane is an insect-transmitted virus that causes congenital abnormalities of the neurological system in ruminants and one of the most potent teratogen viruses affecting cattle, sheep and goats [29, 83]. The incidence of Akabane virus-induced disease is influenced by the species and time of gestation at which infection occurs [29] and by the strain of the virus. Infection in adult cattle has usually no specific signs while infection of pregnant cattle often causes foetal damage, resulting in abortion, stillbirth or various congenital abnormalities [84–86]. A distinct tropism for immature rapidly dividing cells of the foetal central nervous system and skeletal muscle results in direct virus-induced necrotizing encephalomyelitis and polymyositis. The most severe defects are seen after susceptible cows have been infected in earlier gestation. Infection during organogenesis may substantially disrupt structural development in target organs [87] causing arthrogryposis [88], and sometimes also torticollis, kyphosis and scoliosis [29, 84] with associated neurogenic muscle atrophy due to depletion of spinal ventral horn motor neurons, a loss of axons, and depletion of myelin in the lateral and ventral tracts [89]. Calves infected late in pregnancy may be born alive but unable to stand and may have a flaccid paralysis of the limbs, or may be incoordinated and on necropsy show a disseminated encephalomyelitis [90]. These calves have varying degrees of cavitation of cerebral hemispheres. Some calves may be affected with both arthrogryposis and hydranencephaly.

In 1979, Hashiguchi et al. [91] demonstrated that foetal infection in sheep, between 30 and 50 days pregnancy, result in most congenital abnormalities such as ankylosis of the limbs, scoliosis, hydranencephaly, porencephaly, stillbirth with dwarfism and death after birth with dwarfism and weakness. Few, if any, clinical findings are seen after infection in adult animals [84, 91]. In small ruminants, the lesions of arthrogryposis and hydranencephaly are often seen concurrently and are common in the same animals as well as cerebellar hypoplasia, porencephaly, brachygnathia [31, 92]. This type of lesions may or may not be accompanied by inflammation of the central nervous system [31]. Most Akabane-infected lambs or kids are stillborn or die soon after birth.

• Aino virus

Aino virus is a member of the Simbu serogroup of the genus *Orthobunyavirus*, family Bunyaviridae [29, 93]. This virus infection is closely related to the Akabane and SBV infection; therefore, confirmatory diagnosis requires viral detection to differentiate infection between these three viruses [98]. Aino virus is transmitted between animals by insect vectors from *Culicoides* genus mosquitoes [90, 95].

Aino virus infection in adult animals is subclinical, and newborn calves infected can exhibit a wide variety of skeletal and neurological abnormalities [29, 93, 96]. This virus infection is closely related to the Akabane and SBV infection; therefore, confirmatory diagnosis requires viral detection to differentiate infection between these three viruses [94, 98].

In naturally infected pregnant cattle, Aino virus has been associated with abortion [97], stillbirths, premature births and birth congenital malformation, including severe hydranencephaly [98] and/or arthrogryposis [99], unilateral cavitation in the cerebrum, microcephaly and cerebellar hypoplasia [92, 93]. The type of abnormality seen can be related to the time of infection of the foetus [93]: early infection results in hydranencephaly and later infection results in arthrogryposis [99]. Scoliosis [93], sunken eyes, cataracts, maxillary retraction and dental irregularities are also clinical findings. Surviving calves may be weak and can have difficulty suckling or standing. They may also be blind or have poor eyesight. In addition, they may display a variety of neurologic signs, including ataxia, torticollis, tetany, paresis, swimming movements, opisthotonus and circular walking.

• Cache Valley virus

Cache Valley virus (CVV) is a mosquito-borne [100], teratogenic *Bunyavirus* in the *Orthobunyavirus* genus of the Bunyamwera group [1, 101], affecting mainly sheep [106]. Previous studies describing experimental CVV-induced malformations in ovine foetuses showed that the development of foetal lesions is age-dependent. If the virus is inoculated between 28 and 48 days of gestation, foetal death and abortion occur among other lesions [102]; however, foetuses are susceptible at any age demonstrating the tropism of many Orthobunyaviruses for foetal tissues [1, 103]. In general, malformations involve central nervous and musculoskeletal system. Some morphological studies showed necrosis in the central nervous system and skeletal muscle of infected foetuses evaluated after 7–14 days post-infection, and hydrocephalus, micromyelia and muscular loss were observed in infected foetuses after 21–28 days post-infection [1]. Gross pathology of the musculoskeletal system includes arthrogryposis (of one or more limbs), torticollis, scoliosis of the vertebral column and muscular hypoplasia. Central nervous system lesions include hydrancephaly, hydrocephalus, porencephaly, microencephaly, cerebral and cerebellar hypoplasia and micromyelia [1, 103, 104]. Dead embryos and stillborn or mummified lambs are also found [104]. Anasarca is seen, as is oligohydramnios [103]. Limb defects are also due to neurodegenerative changes seen histopathologically as areas of necrosis and loss of paraventricular neutrophils in the brain together with a reduction in the number of motor neurons. Skeletal muscle changes involve poorly developed myotubularmyocytes [104].

• **Chuzan virus**

Chuzan virus is a member of Palymserogroup from genus *Orbivirus*, family Reoviridae, and itis closely related to the Akabane virus and Aino viruses [29, 99]. Chuzan virus is transmitted between animals by insect vectors such as *Culicoides* spp. [105–107] and is considered a teratogen virus once pregnant cows result in foetal congenital abnormalities [96, 108, 109]. Chuzan virus infection in adult animals is subclinical; however, foetal abnormalities in newborn calves infected with Chuzan virus during gestation can exhibit a wide range of skeletal and neurological abnormalities [106]. The most common clinical signs in deformed calves are arthrogryposis, vertebral malformations, brachygnathia inferior and malformations of the central nervous system, including hydranencephaly, porencephaly, hydrocephalus, cerebellar hypoplasia and micromyelia [110].

• **Wesselsbron disease**

Wesselsbron disease is an acute, arthropod-borne infection caused by a flavivirus, member of the Flaviridae family. This virus affects sheep, goats and sporadically cattle [50, 111]. Infection in adult animals and calves is usually subclinical or inapparent [112–114], although in sheep with preexisting liver disease clinical findings can be more expressive and severe. Newborn lambs and kids are most susceptible, and it is often accompanied by a high mortality rate [112, 115]. Outbreaks of congenital abnormalities in foetal or newborn ruminants, musculoskeletal deformities, neonatal deaths [112], abortion in adult animals [31, 50, 112] as well as hydropsamnii [116] in ewes, stillbirths and mummified foetuses [31] have been related. The main lesions found in foetuses are arthrogryposis, brachygnathia inferior, hydranencephaly, hydranencephaly, porencephaly, cerebellar hypoplasia [31], hypoplasia or segmental aplasia of the spinal cord and neurogenic muscular atrophy [116].

Author details

Fernando Esteves[1,2], João Rodrigo Mesquita[1,2,3*], Cármen Nóbrega[1,2], Carla Santos[1,2], António Monteiro[1,2], Rita Cruz[1,2], Helena Vala[1,2,4] and Ana Cláudia Coelho[5]

*Address all correspondence to: jmesquita@esav.ipv.pt

1 Agrarian Superior School of Viseu, Polytechnic Institute of Viseu, Viseu, Portugal

2 Centre for the Study of Education, Technologies and Health (CI&DETS), Polytechnic Institute of Viseu, Viseu, Portugal

3 CIBIO/UP, Research Center in Biodiversity and Genetic Resources/University of Porto, Vairão, Portugal

4 Centre for the Research and Technology of Agro-Environmental and Biological Sciences (CITAB), Vila Real, Portugal

5 Department of Veterinary Sciences, University of Trás-os-Montes and Alto Douro, Vila Real, Portugal

References

[1] Hoffmann B, Scheuch M, Höper D, Jungblut R, Holsteg M, Schirrmeier H, Eschbaumer M, Goller K, Wernike K, Fischer M, Breithaupt A, Mettenleiter T and Lievaart-Peterson K, Luttikholt S, Peperkamp K, Van Den Brom R, Vellema P. (2012). Schmallenberg disease in sheep or goats: Past, present and future. Vet Microbiol. 181, 147-153.

[2] Doceul V, Lara E, Sailleau C, Belbis G, Richardson J, Bréard E, Viarouge C, Dominguez M, Hendrikx P, Calavas D, Desprat A, Languille J, Comtet L, Pourquier P, Eléouët JF. (2013). Epidemiology, molecular virology and diagnostics of Schmallenberg virus, an emerging orthobunyavirus in Europe. Vet Res. 44(1), 31.

[3] Tarlinton R, Daly J, Dunham S, Kydd J. (2012). The challenge of Schmallenberg virus emergence in Europe. Vet J. 194(1), 10-18.

[4] Chen K, Lior P. (2005). Bioinformatics for whole-genome shotgun sequencing of microbial communities. Plos Comput Biol. 1, 106-1012.

[5] Muskens J, Smolenaars A, Van der Poel W, Mars M, Van Wuijckhuise L, Holzhauer M, Kock P. (2012). Diarrhea and loss of production on Dutch dairy farms caused by the Schmallenberg virus. Tijdschr Diergeneeskd. 137(2), 112-115.

[6]   OIE. (2013). Oie technicalfactsheet: Schmallenberg virus. [cited 04 January 2016]. Available from: http://www.oie.int/our-scientific-expertise/specific-information-and-recommendations/schmallenbergvirus/

[7]   Yanase T, Kato M, Aizawa M, Shuto Y, Shirafuji H, Yamakawa M, Tsuda T. (2012). Genetic reassortment between Sathuperi and Shamonda viruses of the genus Ortho-bunyavirus in mature: Implications for their genetic relationship to Schmallenberg virus. Acch. Virol. 157, 1611-1616.

[8]   Elliott RM, Blakqori G, Van Knippenberg IC, Koudriakova E, Li P, McLees A, Shi X, Szemiel AM. (2012). Establishment of a reverse genetics system for Schmallenberg virus, a newly emerged orthobunyavirus in Europe. J Gen Virol. 2013 Apr; 94(Pt 4), 851-859. doi: 10.1099/vir.0.049981-0. Epub 2012 Dec 19.

[9]   Lievaart-Peterson K, Luttikholt S, Peperkamp K, Van den Brom R, Vellema P. (2015). Schmallenberg disease in sheep or goats: Past, present and future. Vet Microbiol. 14;181(1-2), 147-153

[10] Poskin A, Théron L, Hanon JB, Saegerman C, Vervaeke M, Van der Stede Y, De Regge N. (2016). Reconstruction of the Schmallenberg virus epidemic in Belgium: Comple-mentary use of disease surveillance approaches. Vet Microbiol. 183, 50-61.

[11] Esteves F, Mesquita JR, Vala H, Abreu-Silva J, van der Poel WH, Nascimento MS. (2016). Serological evidence for Schmallenberg virus infection in sheep of Portugal. Vector Borne Zoonotic Dis. 16(1), 63-65.

[12] Rasmussen LD, Kirkeby C, Bødker R, Kristensen B, Rasmussen TB, Belsham GJ, Bøtner A. (2014). Rapid spread of Schmallenberg virus-infected biting midges (*Culicoides* spp.) across Denmark in 2012. Transbound Emerg Dis. 61(1), 12-16.

[13] Rasmussen L, Kristensen B, Kirkeby C, Rasmussen T B, Belsham GJ, BØdker R, BØtner A. (2012). Culicoids as vectors of schmallenberg virus. Emerg Infect Dis. 18, 1204-1206.

[14] Elbers AR, Meiswinkel R, Van Weezep E, Kooi EA, van der Poel WH. (2013) Schmal-lenberg virus in Culicoides biting midges in the Netherlands in 2012. Transbound Emerg Dis. 62(3), 339-342.

[15] Ducomble T, Wilking H, Stark K, Takla A, Askar M, Schaade L, Nitsche A, Kurth A. (2012). Lack of evidence for Schmallenberg virus infection in highly exposed persons, Germany, 2012. Emerg Infect Dis. 18(8), 1333-1335.

[16] Herder V, Hansmann F, Wohlsein P, Peters M, Varela M, Palmarini M, Baumgärtner W. (2013). Immunophenotyping of inflammatory cells associated with Schmallenberg virus infection of the central nervous system of ruminants. PLoS One. 7;8(5), e62939.

[17] Wüthrich M, Lechner I, Aebi M, Vögtlin A, Posthaus H, Schüpbach-Regula G, Meylan M. (2016). A case–control study to estimate the effects of acute clinical infection with the Schmallenberg virus on milk yield, fertility and veterinary costs in Swiss dairy herds. Prev Vet Med. 126:54-65.

[18] Afonso, A, Abrahantes, JC, Conraths, F, Veldhuis, A, Elbers, A, Roberts, H Richardson, J. (2014). The Schmallenberg virus epidemic in Europe—2011–2013. Prev Vet Med. 116, 391-403.

[19] Parsonson IM, Della-Porta AJ, Snowdon WA. (1977). Congenital abnormalities in newborn lambs after infection of pregnant sheep with Akabane virus. Infect Immun. 15(1), 254-262.

[20] Coetzee P, Stokstad M, Venter EH, Myrmel M, Van Vuuren M. (2012). Bluetongue: A historical and epidemiological perspective with the emphasis on South Africa. Virol J. 9, 198.

[21] MacLachlan NJ. (1994). The pathogenesis and immunology of bluetongue virus infection of ruminants. Comp Immunol Microbiol Infect Dis. Aug-Nov; 17(3-4), 197-206.

[22] Osborne CJ, Mayo CE, Mullens BA, McDermott EG, Gerry AC, Reisen WK, MacLachlan NJ. (2015). Lack of evidence for laboratory and natural vertical transmission of blue-tongue virus in Culicoidessonorensis (Diptera: Ceratopogonidae). J Med Entomol. 52(2), 274-277.

[23] Mayo CE, Gardner IA, Mullens BA, Barker CM, Gerry AC, Guthrie AJ, MacLachlan NJ. (2012). Anthropogenic and meteorological factors influence vector abundance and prevalence of bluetongue virus infection of dairy cattle in California. Vet Microbiol. Mar 23; 155(2-4), 158-164. doi: 10.1016/j.vetmic.2011.08.029.

[24] Caporale M, Di Gialleonorado L, Janowicz A, Wilkie G, Shaw A, Savini G, Van Rijn PA, Mertens P, Di Ventura M, Palmarini M. (2014). Virus and host factors affecting the clinical outcome of bluetongue virus infection. J Virol. 88(18), 10399-10411.

[25] Maclachlan NJ, Drew CP, Darpel KE, Worwa G. (2009). The pathology and pathogenesis of bluetongue. J Comp Pathol. Jul; 141(1), 1-16.

[26] van Wuijckhuise L, Dercksen D, Muskens J, de Bruijn J, Scheepers M, Vrouenraets R. (2006). Bluetongue in the Netherlands; description of the first clinical cases and differential diagnosis. Common symptoms just a little different and in too many herds. Tijdschr Diergeneeskd. 131(18), 649-654

[27] Najarnezhad V, Rajae M. (2013). Seroepidemiology of bluetongue disease in small ruminants of north-east of Iran. Asian Pac J Trop Biomed. 3(6), 492-495.

[28] Darpel KE, Batten CA, Veronesi E, Williamson S, Anderson P, Dennison M, Clifford S, Smith C, Philips L, Bidewell C, Bachanek-Bankowska K, Sanders A, Bin-Tarif A, Wilson AJ, Gubbins S, Mertens PP, Oura CA, Mellor PS. (2009). Transplacental transmission of bluetongue virus 8 in cattle, UK.Emerg Infect Dis. 15(12), 2025-2028.

[29] Agerholm JS, Hewicker-Trautwein M, Peperkamp K, Windsor PA. (2015) Virus-induced congenital malformations in cattle. Acta Vet Scand. Sep 24; 57, 54.

[30] Wilson WC, Bawa B, Drolet BS, Lehiy C, Faburay B, Jasperson DC, Reister L, Gaudreault NN, Carlson J, Ma W, Morozov I, McVey DS, Richt JA. (2014). Evaluation of lamb and calf responses to Rift Valley fever MP-12 vaccination. Vet Microbiol. Aug 6; 172(1-2), 44-50.

[31] Javanbakht J, Mardjanmehr SH, Tavasoly A, Nazemshirazi MH. (2014). Neuropathological microscopic features of abortions induced by Bunyavirus / or Flavivirus infections. Diagn Pathol. 9, 223

[32] Eschbaumer M, Wernike K, Batten CA, Savini G, Edwards L, Di Gennaro A, Teodori L, Oura CA, Beer M, Hoffmann B. (2012). Epizootic hemorrhagic disease virus serotype 7 in European cattle and sheep: Diagnostic considerations and effect of previous BTV exposure. Vet Microbiol. 159(3-4), 298-306.

[33] Temizel EM, Yesilbag K, Batten C, Senturk S, Maan NS, Mertens PPC. (2009). Epizootic hemorrhagic disease in cattle, western Turkey. Emerg Infect Dis. 15, 2.

[34] Brodie SJ, Bardsley KD, Diem K, Mecham JO, Norelius SE, Wilson WC. (1988). Epizootic hemorrhagic disease: Analysis of tissues by amplification and in situ hybridization reveals widespread orbivirus infection at low copy numbers. J Virol. 72(5), 3863-3871.

[35] Cêtre-Sossah C, Roger M, Sailleau C, Rieau L, Zientara S, Bréard E, Viarouge C, Beral M, Esnault O, Cardinale E. (2014). Epizootic haemorrhagic disease virus in Reunion Island: Evidence for the circulation of a new serotype and associated risk factors. Vet Microbiol. Jun 4; 170(3-4), 383-390.

[36] Maclachlan NJ, Guthrie A (2010). Re-emergence of bluetongue, African horse sickness, and other Orbivirus diseases. Vet Res. 41(6): 35.

[37] Maclachlan NJ, Zientara S, Savini G, Daniels PW. (2015). Epizootic haemorrhagic disease. Rev Sci Tech. Aug; 34(2), 341-351

[38] Anbalagan S, Hause BM. (2014). Characterization of epizootic hemorrhagic disease virus from a bovine with clinical disease with high nucleotide sequence identity to white-tailed deer isolates. Arch Virol. Oct; 159(10), 2737-2740.

[39] OIE Terrestrial Manual. (2014). Epizootic haemorrhagic disease. [cited 04 January 2016]. Available from: http://www.oie.int/fileadmin/Home/fr/Health_standards/tahm/ 2.01.04b_EHD.pdf.

[40] Longjam N, Deb R, Sarmah AK, Tayo T, Awachat VB, Saxena VK. (2011). A brief review on diagnosis of foot-and-mouth disease of livestock: Conventional to molecular tools. Vet Med Int. 2011, 905768.

[41] Grubman MJ, Baxt B. (2004). Foot-and-mouth disease. Clin Microbiol Rev. April; 17(2), 465-493.

[42] Doll K. (2001). Clinical picture and differential diagnosis of foot and mouth disease in cattle. Dtsch Tierarztl Wochenschr. 108(12), 494-498.

[43] Lyons NA, Alexander N, Stärk K, Dulu TD, Rushton J, Fine PEM. (2015). Impact of foot-and-mouth disease on mastitis and culling on a large-scale dairy farm in Kenya. Vet Res. 46(1), 41

[44] Knight-Jones TJD, Rushtonb J. (2013). The economic impacts of foot and mouth disease — What are they, how big are they and where do they occur? Prev Vet Med. 1;112(3-4), 161-173.

[45] Weir E. (2001). Foot-and-mouth disease in animals and humans. CMAJ. 1;164(9), 1338.

[46] Kitching RP, Hughes GJ. (2002). Clinical variation in foot and mouth disease: Sheep and goats. Rev Sci Tech. Dec; 21(3), 505-512.

[47] Donaldson AI, Alexandersen S. (2002). Predicting the spread of foot and mouth disease by airborne virus. Rev Sci Tech. Dec; 21(3), 569-575.

[48] Meyer RF, Knudsen RC. (2001). Foot-and-mouth disease: a review of the virus and the symptoms. J Environ Health. 64(4):21–3.

[49] Ridpath JF. (2010). Bovine viral diarrhea virus: Global status. Vet Clin North Am Food Anim Pract. Mar; 26(1), 105-121.

[50] Ali H, Ali AA, Atta MS, Cepica A. (2011). Common, emerging, vector-borne and infrequent abortogenic virus infections of cattle. Transbound Emerg Dis. 59(1), 11-25.

[51] Deregt D, Loewen KG. (1995). Bovine viral diarrhea virus: Biotypes and disease. Can Vet J. 36(6), 371-378.

[52] Grooms DL. (2004). Reproductive consequences of infection with bovine viral diarrhea virus. Vet Clin North Am Food Anim Pract. Mar; 20(1), 5-19.

[53] Houe H. (1995). Epidemiology of bovine viral diarrhea virus. Vet Clin North Am Food Anim Pract. Nov; 11(3), 521-547.

[54] Hessman BE, Sjeklocha DB, Fulton RW, Ridpath JF, Johnson BJ, McElroy DR. (2012). Acute bovine viral diarrhea associated with extensive mucosal lesions, high morbidity, and mortality in a commercial feedlot. J Vet Diagn Invest. 24, 397.

[55] Goens DS. (2002). The evolution of bovine viral diarrhea: A review. Can Vet J. Dec; 43(12), 946-954.

[56] Meyling A, Jensen AM. (1988). Transmission of bovine virus diarrhoea virus (BVDV) by artificial insemination (AI) with semen from a persistently-infected bull. Vet Microbiol. Jun; 17(2), 97-105.

[57] Niskanen R, Lindberg A. (2003). Transmission of bovine viral diarrhoea virus by unhygienic vaccination procedures, ambient air, and from contaminated pens. Vet J. Mar; 165(2), 125-130.

[58] Nettleton PF, Gilray JA, Russo P, Dlissi E. (1998). Border disease of sheep and goats. Vet Res. May-Aug; 29(3-4), 327-340.

[59] García-Pérez AL, Minguijón E, Estévez L, Barandika JF, Aduriz G, Juste RA, Hurtado A. (2009). Clinical and laboratorial findings in pregnant ewes and their progeny infected with Border disease virus (BDV-4 genotype). Res Vet Sci. Apr; 86(2), 345-352.

[60] Nettleton PF. (1987). Pathogenesis and epidemiology of border disease. Ann Rech Vet. 18(2), 147-155.

[61] Lim CF, Carnegie PR. (1984). A survey of hairy shaker disease (border disease, hypo-myelinogenesiscongenita) in sheep. Aust Vet J. Jun; 61(6), 174-177.

[62] Osburn BI, Castrucci G. (1991). Diaplacental infections with ruminant pestiviruses. Arch Virol Suppl. 3, 71-78.

[63] Terpstra C. (1980). Border disease: a persistent virus infection in sheep (author's transl). Tijdschr Diergeneeskd. Aug 15; 105(16), 650-656.

[64] Lemaire M, Meyer G, Baranowski E, Schynts F, Wellemans G, Kerkhofs, Thiry E. (2000). Production of Bovine herpesvirus type 1-seronegative latent carriers by administration of a live-attenuated vaccine in passively immunized calves. J Clin Microbiol. Nov; 38(11), 4233-4238.

[65] Thiry J, Keuser V, Muylkens B, Meurens F, Gogev S, Vanderplasschen A, Thiry E. (2006). Ruminant alphaherpesviruses related to bovine herpesvirus 1. Vet Res. Mar-Apr; 37(2), 169-190.

[66] Furuoka H, Izumida N, Horiuchi M, Osame S, Matsui T. (1995). Bovine herpesvirusmeningoencephalitis association with infectious bovine rhinotracheitis (IBR) vaccine. Acta Neuropathol. 90(6), 565-571

[67] Engels M1, Ackermann M. (1996). Pathogenesis of ruminant herpesvirus infections. Vet Microbiol. 1996 Nov; 53(1-2), 3-15.

[68] Jones C1, Chowdhury S. (2007). A review of the biology of bovine herpesvirus type 1 (BHV-1), its role as a cofactor in the bovine respiratory disease complex and development of improved vaccines. Anim Health Res Rev. Dec; 8(2), 187-205.

[69] Nuotio L, Neuvonen E, Hyytiäinen M. (2007). Epidemiology and eradication of infectious bovine rhinotracheitis/infectious pustularvulvovaginitis (IBR/IPV) virus in Finland. Acta Vet Scand. 49(1), 3

[70] Grewal AS, Wells R. (1986). Vulvovaginitis of goats due to a herpesvirus. Aust Vet J. Mar; 63(3), 79-82.

[71] Chénier S, Montpetit C, Hélie P. (2004). Caprine herpesvirus-1 abortion storm in a goat herd in Quebec. Can Vet J. Mar; 45(3), 241-243.

[72] Ikegami T, Makino S. (2011). The pathogenesis of Rift Valley fever. Viruses. 3, 493-519; doi: 10.3390/v3050493

[73] Chamchod F, Cosner C, Cantrell RS, Beier JC, Ruan S. (2015). Transmission dynamics of Rift Valley fever virus: Effects of live and killed vaccines on epizootic outbreaks and enzootic maintenance. Front Microbiol. 6, 1568.

[74] Lutomiah J, Omondi D, Masiga D, Mutai C, Mireji PO, Ongus J, Linthicum KJ, Sang R. (2014). Blood meal analysis and virus detection in blood-fed mosquitoes collected during the 2006–2007 Rift Valley fever outbreak in Kenya. Vector Borne Zoonotic Dis. 14(9), 656–364.

[75] LaBeaud D, Pfeil F, Traylor Z, Hise G, Kazura JW, Gildengorin G, Muiruri S, Muchiri EM, King CH. (2015). Factors associated with severe human Rift Valley fever in Sangailu, Garissa County, Kenya. PLOS Negl Trop Dis. 12;9(3):e0003548.

[76] Munyua P, Murithi RM, Wainwright S, Githinji J, Hightower A, Mutonga D, Macharia J, Ithondeka PM, Musaa J, Breiman RF, Bloland P, Njenga MK. (2010). Rift Valley fever outbreak in Livestock in Kenya, 2006–2007. Am J Trop Med Hyg. 5;83(2 Suppl), 58-64.

[77] Bakhshesh M, Abdollahi D. (2015). Bovine Ephemeral fever in Iran: Diagnosis, isolation and molecular characterization. J Arthropod Borne Dis. 9(2), 195-203.

[78] Trinidad L, Blasdell KR, Joubert DA, Davis SS, Melville L, Kirkland PD, Coulibaly F, Holmes EC, Walke PJ. (2014). Evolution of bovine ephemeral fever virus in the Australian Episystem. J Virol. 88(3), 1525-1535.

[79] Nandi S, Negi BS. (1999). Bovine ephemeral fever: A review. Comp Immunol Microbiol Infect Dis. Apr; 22(2), 81-91.

[80] Kirkland PD (2002). Akabane and bovine ephemeral fever virus infections. Vet Clin North Am Food Anim Pract. Nov; 18(3), 501-514, viii-ix.

[81] Walker PJ (2005). Bovine ephemeral fever in Australia and the world. Curr Top Microbiol Immunol. 292, 57-80.

[82] Liao YK, Inaba Y, Li NJ, Chain CY, Lee SL, Liou PP. (1998). Epidemiology of bovine ephemeral fever virus infection in Taiwan. Microbiol Res. Nov; 153(3), 289-295.

[83] Beer M, Conraths FJ, van der Poel WH. (2013). 'Schmallenberg virus' – A novel orthobunyavirus emerging in Europe. Epidemiol Infect. Jan; 141(1), 1-8.

[84] Oluwayelu DO, Aiki-Raji CO, Umeh EC, Mustapha SO, Adebiyi AI. (2016). Serological investigation of Akabane virus infection in cattle and sheep in Nigeria. Adv Virol. 2016, 2936082. Published online 2016 January 26.

[85] Kirkland PD. (2015). Akabane virus infection. Rev Sci Tech. Aug; 34(2), 403-410.

[86] Elhassan AM, Mansour MEA, Shamon AAA, El Hussein AM. (2014). A serological survey of Akabane virus infection in cattle in Sudan. ISRN Vet Sci. 2014, 123904. Published online 2014 January 21.

[87] Charles JA. (1994). Akabane virus. Vet Clin North Am Food Anim Pract. Nov; 10(3), 525-546.

[88] Kurogi H, Inaba Y, Takahashi E, Sato K, Satoda K. (1977). Congenital abnormalities in newborn calves after inoculation of pregnant cows with Akabane virus. Infect Immun. 17(2), 338-343.

[89] Gundlach AL, Grabara CS, Johnston GA, Harper PA. (1990). Receptor alterations associated with spinal motoneuron degeneration in bovine Akabane disease. Ann Neurol. May; 27(5), 513-519.

[90] Kono R, Hirata M, Kaji M, Goto Y, Ikeda S, Yanase T, Kato T, Tanaka S, Tsutsui T, Imada T, Yamakawa M. (2008). Bovine epizootic encephalomyelitis caused by Akabane virus in southern Japan. BMC Vet Res. 4, 20.

[91] Hashiguchi Y, Nanba K, Kumagai T. (1979). Congenital abnormalities in newborn lambs following Akabane virus infection in pregnant ewes. Natl Inst Anim Health Q, 19(1-2), 1-11.

[92] Haughey KG, Hartley WJ, Della-Porta AJ, Murray MD. (1988). Akabane disease in sheep. Aust Vet J. May; 65(5), 136-140.

[93] Tsuda T, Yoshida K, Ohashi S, Yanase T, Sueyoshi M, Kamimura S, Misumi K, Hamana K, Sakamoto H, Yamakawa M. (2004). Arthrogryposis, hydranencephaly and cerebellar hypoplasia syndrome in neonatal calves resulting from intrauterine infection with Aino virus. Vet Res. 35(5), 531-538.

[94] Lee JH, Seo HJ, Park JY, Kim SH, Cho YS, Kim YJ, Cho IS, Jeoung HY. (2015). Detection and differentiation of Schmallenberg, Akabane and Aino viruses by one-step multiplex reverse-transcriptase quantitative PCR assay. BMC Vet Res. 24;11, 270.

[95] Kim YH, Kweon CH, Tark DS, Lim SI, Yang DK, Hyun BH, Song JY, Hur W, Park SC. (2011). Development of inactivated trivalent vaccine for the teratogenic Aino, Akabane and Chuzan viruses. Biologicals. May; 39(3), 152-157.

[96] Hechinger S, Wernike K, Beer M. (2013). Evaluating the protective efficacy of a trivalent vaccine containing Akabane virus, Aino virus and Chuzan virus against Schmallenberg virus infection. Vet Res. 5;44, 114.

[97] Uchinuno Y, Noda Y, Ishibashi K, Nagasue S, Shirakawa H, Nagano M, Ohe R. (1998). Isolation of Aino virus from an aborted bovine fetus. J Vet Med Sci. 60(10), 1139-1140.

[98] Kitano Y, Yamashita S, Makinoda K. (1994). A congenital abnormality of calves, suggestive of a new type of arthropod-borne virus infection. J Comp Pathol. Nov; 111(4), 427-437.

[99] Noda Y, Uchinuno Y, Shirakawa H, Nagasue S, Nagano N, Ohe R, Narita M. (1998). Aino virus antigen in brain lesions of a naturally aborted bovine fetus. Vet Pathol. 35(5), 409-411.

[100] Andreadis TG, Armstrong PM, Anderson JF, Main AJ. (2014). Spatial-temporal analysis of Cache Valley virus (Bunyaviridae: Orthobunyavirus) infection in anopheline and culicine mosquitoes (Diptera: Culicidae) in the northeastern United States, 1997-2012. Vector Borne Zoonotic Dis. 14(10), 763-773.

[101] Edwards JF. (1994). Cache Valley virus. Vet Clin North Am Food Anim Pract. Nov; 10(3), 515-524.

[102] Rodrigues Hoffmann A, Dorniak P, Filant J, Dunlap KA, Bazer FW, de la Concha-Bermejillo A, Welsh CJ, Varner P, Edwards JF. (2013). Ovine fetal immune response to Cache Valley virus infection. J Virol. 87(10), 5586-5592.

[103] Chung SI, Livingston CW Jr, Edwards JF, Gauer BB, Collisson EW. (1990). Congenital malformations in sheep resulting from in utero inoculation of Cache Valley virus. Am J Vet Res. Oct; 51(10), 1645-1648.

[104] Edwards JF, Karabatsos N, Collisson EW, de la Concha Bermejillo A. (1997). Ovine fetal malformations induced by in utero inoculation with Main Drain, San Angelo, and LaCrosse viruses. Emerg Infect Dis. 3(2), 195-197.

[105] Lim SI, Kweon CH, Tark DS, Kim SH, Yang DK. (2007). Sero-survey on Aino, Akabane, Chuzan, bovine ephemeral fever and Japanese encephalitis virus of cattle and swine in Korea. J Vet Sci. Mar; 8(1), 45-49.

[106] Kim YH, Kweon CH, Tark DS, Lim SI, Yang DK, Hyun BH, Song JY, Hur W, Park SC. (2011). Development of inactivated trivalent vaccine for the teratogenic Aino, Akabane and Chuzan viruses .Biologicals. May; 39(3), 152-157.

[107] Ohashi S, Yoshida K, Yanase T, Kato T, Tsuda T. (2004). Simultaneous detection of bovine arboviruses using single-tube multiplex reverse transcription-polymerase chain reaction. J Virol Methods. 1;120(1), 79-85.

[108] Oberst RD. (1993). Viruses as teratogens. The veterinary clinics of North America. Food Anim Pract. 9(1), 23-31

[109] Miura Y, Kubo M, Goto Y, Kono Y. (1990). Hydranencephaly-cerebellar hypoplasia in a newborn calf after infection of its dam with Chuzan virus. Nihon Juigaku Zasshi. Aug; 52(4), 689-694.

[110] Goto Y, Miura Y, Kono Y. (1988). Serologic evidence for the etiologic role of Chuzan virus in an epizootic of congenital abnormalities with hydranencephaly-cerebellar hypoplasia syndrome of calves in Japan. Am J Vet Res. Dec; 49(12), 2026-2029.

[111] Blackburn NK, Swanepoel R. (1980). An investigation of flavivirus infections of cattle in Zimbabwe Rhodesia with particular reference to Wesselsbron virus. J Hyg (Lond). 85(1), 1-33.

[112] Mushi EZ, Binta MG, Raborokgwe M. (1998). Wesselsbron disease virus associated with abortions in goats in Botswana. J Vet Diagn Invest. 10(2), 191.

[113] Coetzer JA, Theodoridis A. (1982). Clinical and pathological studies in adult sheep and goats experimentally infected with Wesselsbron disease virus. Onderstepoort J Vet Res. 49(1), 19-22.

[114] Coetzer JA, Theodoridis A, Herr S, Kritzinger L. (1979). Wesselsbron disease: A cause of congenital porencephaly and cerebellar hypoplasia in calves. Onderstepoort J Vet Res. 46(3), 165-169

[115] Jupp PG, Kemp A. (1998). Studies on an outbreak of Wesselsbron virus in the Free State Province, South Africa. J Am Mosq Control Assoc. 14(1), 40-45

[116] Coetzer JA, Barnard BJ. (1977). Hydropsamnii in sheep associated with hydranence-phaly and arthrogryposis with Wesselsbron disease and Rift Valley fever viruses as aetiological agents. Onderstepoort J Vet Res. Jun; 44(2), 119-126.

Chapter 4

Epidemiology and Emergence of Schmallenberg Virus Part 2: Pathogenesis and Risk of Viral Spread

Fernando Esteves, João Rodrigo Mesquita,
Cármen Nóbrega, Carla Santos, António Monteiro,
Rita Cruz, Helena Vala and Ana Cláudia Coelho

Additional information is available at the end of the chapter

http://dx.doi.org/10.5772/64742

Abstract

Schmallenberg virus (SBV) is a novel Orthobunyavirus causing mild clinical signs in cows and malformations in aborted and neonatal ruminants in Europe. SBV belongs to the family Bunyaviridae and is transmitted by biting midges. This new virus was identified for the first time in blood samples of cows in the city of Schmallenberg in North-Rhine Westphalia in November 2011. Since then, the virus spread to several European countries. Here, we describe the pathogenesis and the risk of viral spread in the Portuguese territory.

Keywords: Schmallenberg virus, emerging infections, epidemiology

1. Pathogenesis

The knowledge of Schmallenberg virus (SBV) pathogeny will allow to achieve a better understanding of its most obvious expression, reflected in their striking lesional pattern; however, until now, the pathogenic features of SBV are not well understood. Current assumptions about SBV pathogenesis in ruminants are frequently based on findings described for Akabane virus (AKAV), which, similar to SBV, causes in aborted or stillborn neonatal ruminants, arthrogryposis and hydranencephaly syndrome (AHS) [1].

The tropism of SBV to the central nervous system (CNS) is already well described in the literature, associated with several congenital malformations, being the most notorious in the

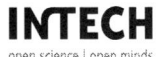

brain [2]. However, taking into consideration the results obtained by Balseiro et al. [3], regarding the presence of the virus in several tissues of naturally infected calves, SBV could also have tropism to other organs and tissues, namely muscle, skeletal and cardiac, spleen, placenta and umbilical cord [3].

As referred, SBV infection during gestational period affects the foetus, through a vertical transplacental transmission. The development of teratogenic defects and its severity is directly related with gestational time (GT) at the moment of infection and, consequently, neuronal cells development in the CNS, which are the SBV target [2, 3].

The severity of lesions in the CNS is also dependent of the foetal immune system development, characterized by cellular population of the thymus and lymph nodes and the production of antibodies, which in bovines occurs between days 40 and 175 of GT and in the lamb starts 19 days post gestation and lasts until 115 days after conception and depends also of the foetal CNS vulnerability (well defined in the cow as the period between days 60 and 180 of GT) [1, 2].

Thus, the severity of lesions in the brain and spinal cord depends on the complexity of the interaction between foetal neurogenesis, immunocompetency, virulence of the viral strain, intensity and time of infection [1–3].

If maternal infection occurs in early gestational period, before the foetus becomes immuno-competent (between the 90th and the 180th day of GT in cow; between the 25th and 50th day in sheep), severe dysplastic CNS lesions, including a distinctive micromyelia, without evidence of inflammation are described, as well as abortion, stillborn and congenital malformations, with no detectable viral RNA and antigen [2, 4, 5].

Infection in the first month of gestation could probably cause embryonic death and subsequent resorption or abortion, only proven by repeat oestrus and matings, observed by farmers and shepherds [4].

If maternal infection occurs in the late gestational period (after 180th day of GT in cow; after 50th day in sheep), inflammation—nonsuppurative polioencephalomyelitis (lymphohistio-cytic) or meningoencephalomyelitis—can be present due to viral antigen recognition by the foetal immune system, with detectable viral RNA and antigen [1, 2, 4, 5].

Probably due to the rapid organogenesis consequent to the shorter GT in sheep (GT of 150–155 days), brain and spinal cord malformation are more severe in lambs than in calves [5]. As well as most viral infections, transplacental transmission could not result in notorious placentitis and most malformed newborns are stillborn at term [2].

1.1. CNS congenital malformations

The association of Schmallenberg virus with a range of congenital malformations, mostly in the CNS, is well known [2]. The brain is the most frequent target, but cerebellar and spinal cord defects are also referred by several authors [5]. The predominant malformations observed in the CNS of both lambs and calves are hydranencephaly, porencephaly, hydrocephalus, microencephaly, cerebellar hypoplasia and mild-to-marked dysplasia of the cerebellum, brain stem and spinal cord [4, 6].

According to Peperkamp et al. [5], defects occurring in the cerebrum might range from slight to moderate dysplasia, including microencephaly, porencephaly, hydrocephalus and lack of gyri (lissencephaly), to fully developed hydranencephaly.

Porencephaly refers to cystic fluid-filled cavities in the brain tissue, which communicate with the ventricular system, and is usually described as the cavitation of the cerebral hemispheres. One study performed by Herder et al. [1] revealed that the temporal and parietal lobes are more frequently affected, usually in a bilateral-symmetrical matter. Furthermore, porencephaly might be present in both temporal and parietal lobes, in a condition named multicystic encephalopathy.

Hydranencephaly is characterized by the destruction of brain hemispheres, many times with a complete or almost complete replacement of the cortex by cerebrospinal fluid, surrounded by a thin, almost transparent, membranous sac.

Cerebellar hypoplasia is one of the most frequently referred malformations in the CNS of SBV-infected animals, and, both in lambs and in calves, various degrees of cerebellar dysplasia might be present, even in animals presenting a normal cerebrum [5].

Morphologic alterations of the spinal cord are observed as a decrease in the cross-sectional area of the spinal cord, or micromyelia. This malformation is characterized by neuronal loss in the ventral horns, and is apparently positively correlated with the magnitude of musculoskeletal deformities [5].

Histologically, the described malformations might be accompanied by the presence or absence of inflammation, including encephalomyelitis, lymphohistiocytic meningoencephalomyelitis and glial nodules. Microscopic lesions include rarefaction and cavitation, degeneration, necrosis and loss of neurons, as well as mild to severe, diffuse astrogliosis and/or microgliosis [1, 7].

1.2. Other lesions (musculoskeletal)

Malformed newborns presented underweight due to the underdevelopment of body mass, skeletal muscles and variable severity of malformations. Frequently, bones undergo normal development but vertebral malformations and arthrogryposis occur due to the imbalance in foetal muscular activity, secondary to the loss of neurons in the brain and spinal cord and demyelination, affecting descending tracts in the ventral spinal cord white matter, ventral horn motor neurons in the spinal cord grey matter and ventral spinal nerve roots [2, 4, 8].

The lack of innervation, by lower motor neuron, to the skeletal muscle motor units prevents its normal development, resulting in muscular hypoplasia. Neuronal bilateral loss in cervical and lumbar intumescences causes bilateral arthrogryposis, and unilateral neuronal loss causes unilateral arthrogryposis [4, 5].

This neuronal loss in spinal cord could be grossly visible in severely affected cases, as a small dorsoventral flattened spinal cord, designated by micromyelia and, consequently, results in denervation of the axial and appendicular musculature with the failure of normal skeletal muscle development, resulting in the lesions of vertebral column malformations and arthrogryposis [2].

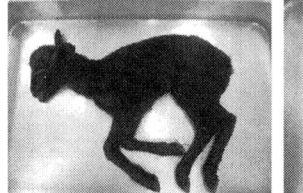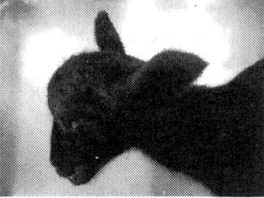

Figure 1. Newborn lamb with 6 days revealing prognathism and kyphosis.

Therefore, vertebral column malformations, namely torticollis, scoliosis and kyphosis (**Figure 1**) of the thoracic vertebral column, mostly combined with arthrogryposis are consequent to dysplastic CNS lesions and represent the most visible gross lesions [2]. Scoliosis, kyphoscoliosis and kyphosis without torticollis are less frequent and vertebral column malformations without arthrogryposis are rare (**Table 1**) [2].

Frequency	Arthrogryposis	Vertebral column malformations			
		Torticollis	Scoliosis	Kyphosis	Torticollis
Frequent	x	x	x	x	x
Less frequent			x	x	
Rare		x	x	x	x

Table 1. Most visible gross lesions.

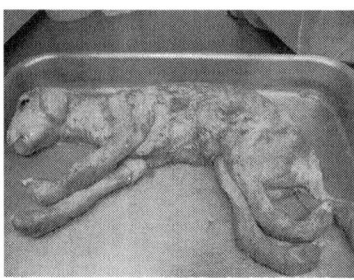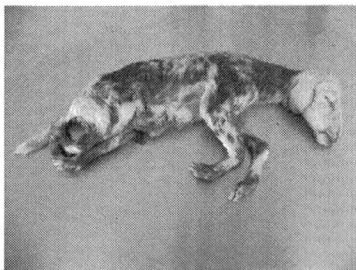

Figure 2. Stillborn lambs with severe arthrogryposis multiplex congenital affecting the four limbs.

The most frequent lesion observed in the limbs is the arthrogryposis multiplex congenital affecting the four limbs, symmetric and bilaterally (**Figures 2–4**), often accompanied by vertebral column malformations, as referred. Arthrogryposis could range from different severities, affecting only the forelimbs (uni- or bilaterally) or only the hindlimbs (uni- or bilaterally; rarely) (**Table 2**) [2, 5].

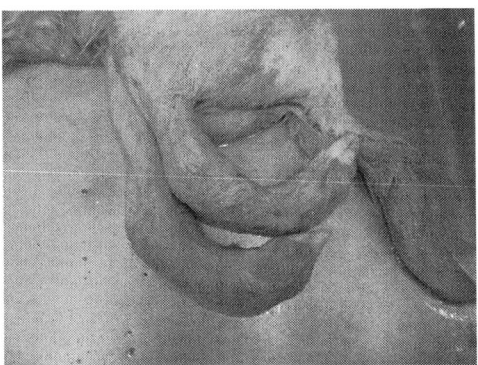

Figure 3. Arthrogryposis. Note the severe curving of joints.

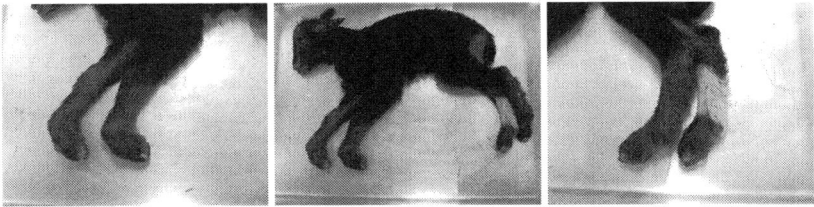

Figure 4. Newborn kid with three revealing arthrogryposis affecting only forelimbs bilaterally.

	Forelimb right	Forelimb left	Hindlimb right	Hindlimb left
Frequent	x	x	x	x
Less frequent	x	x		
Rare			x	x

Table 2. Frequency of arthrogryposis.

The histopathology of skeletal muscles of arthrogrypotic limbs revealed hypoplasia of striated muscular tissue (severe reduction of muscle diameter) and myofibrillar hypoplasia, reflecting the extent of dysplastic spinal cord with neuronal loss in the cervical and lumbar intumescences [2, 4, 5]. Other musculoskeletal histopathologic lesions described include atrophy and loss of skeletal muscle mass (especially in the limbs and neck) (**Figure 5**), with the presence of fibrous or adipose tissue, as well as the depletion of fat deposits [5, 9].

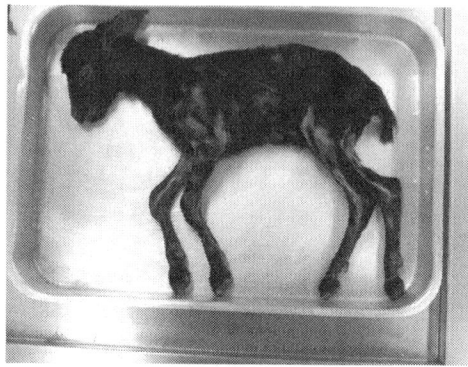

Figure 5. Newborn kid with 6 days revealing the loss of skeletal muscle mass.

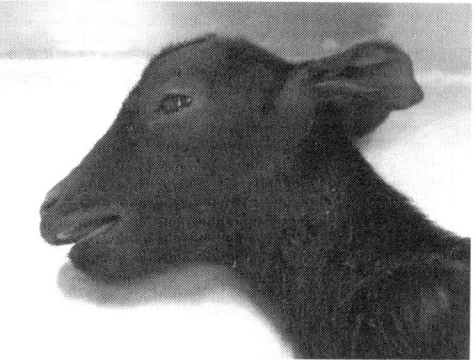

Figure 6. Newborn kid with 3 days revealing brachygnathia.

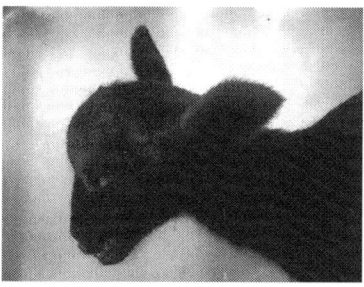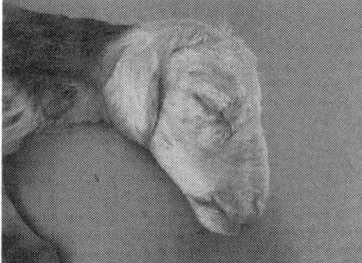

Figure 7. Stillborn lamb with prognathism.

Abnormal flattened skull with cranial vault reduced by thickened frontal, parietal and occipital bones was described [5]. Flattened ribcage could also be present, consequently to malformations of the thoracic vertebral column, as well as lordosis of the thoracolumbar part of the vertebral column [2].

Lesions of brachygnathia (**Figure 6**) and prognathism (**Figure 7**) are described in the consulted literature [5, 9].

Peperkamp et al. [5] reported hypoplasia of the lung lobes in ruminants affected with thoracic malformation but in other organs analysed, such as urinary bladder, thyroid gland, liver, spleen, heart muscle and vessels, uterus, ovaries, testes, peripheral nerves, placenta, oesophagus, abomasum, small and large intestine, pancreas, adrenal glands, celiac ganglion, trachea, skin, tongue and adipose tissue, no significant histopathological lesions were present [5, 9].

1.3. Characterization of inflammatory infiltrates

Inflammatory changes of the brain and meninges are more frequent in small ruminants than in calves, and are characterized by lymphohistiocytic perivascular cuffs with parenchymal T cells, B cells and microglia/macrophages. The CD3-positive T cells are the dominant cellular group. CD79α-positive B cells are also found, but on a lesser extent and CD68-positive microglia/macrophages are less often detected [1].

1.4. Challenges in differential diagnosis

Taking into account the most prominent lesion of CNS congenital malformations, in ruminants, the first and most important challenge in the differential diagnosis (DD) is ruling out other viral-induced congenital malformations in ruminants, including bovine virus diarrhoea virus (BVDV), Border disease virus (BDV), blue tongue virus (BTV), Akabane virus, Aino virus (AV) and Cache Valley virus (CVV) [2, 5].

Also, molecular and serological diagnosis becomes more difficult when the infection of SBV occurs in early gestational period (aggravated in cows where the total GT is larger than sheep) for having more time to develop an effective immune response (foetal lambs have its immune system completely immunocompetent at mid-gestation, at the 90th day of GT) and performs the viral clearance in seropositive offspring, which could make them negative to the virus [4, 5]. Moreover, malformations in CNS and musculoskeletal system are frequently caused by teratogenic and genetic defects, as well as a significant number of inherited congenital syndromes that closely resemble SBV lesions, such as arthrogryposis multiplex congenital syndrome, arachnomelia, both with arthrogryposis [2]. Also, rare non-viral congenital syndromes can occur, such as congenital myoclonus, Perosomus elumbis, Cyclopia and none fragility described in bovine.

Unlike clinical signs, discrete, non-specific and variable, the lesions described above have a dramatic and showy expression, could be easily recognized by clinicians but none are pathognomonic for SBV, despite its great diagnostic value (**Table 3**). It is then extremely difficult to obtain a precise and definitive aetiological diagnosis [2, 5].

	SBV	BTV	BVDV and BDV	AKAV
Cerebral defects	Yes or no (less common in cow)	Yes	Yes	Yes in early GT
Spinal cord lesions with arthrogryposis	Yes	No	No	Yes in late GT
Vertebral malformations	Yes	No	No	No (rare)

Table 3. The value of congenital malformations in the DD of viral-induced congenital malformations.

Therefore, definitive diagnosis requires systematic necropsies, with the examination of the brain and spinal cord, which could be done in the field but the ideal practice would be the recourse to a specialty laboratory to obtain diagnostic accuracy and specificity namely the pathology laboratory, once the diagnosis could not be exclusively done based only in gross lesions, even if arthrogryposis is present [2, 10] and require histopathology of the entire CNS whose collection should be complete, which is labour intensive and requires specific material to be performed (**Figure 8**).

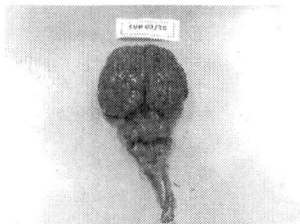

Figure 8. Complete collection of CNS of a newborn kid with 3 days.

Pathological diagnosis must be complemented by molecular genetics, serological and virological diagnosis [2, 3].

Dissemination of information about the disease, especially in the moment of the entrance into a given country, is crucial to alert professionals about the emergence of outbreaks, the data registration for each suspect or compatible case being crucial, as proposed in **Table 4**. In this registration, it is mandatory to include the date of occurrence, season and geographic region information, to relate with vector activity, since as in the winter, with too low temperatures for the vector activity, SBV may be soon ruled out [2].

Collection date (season)	Herd code	Parish	Municipality	Earmark mother	Species	Race	Gender	Abortion	Perinatal death	Stillborn
								Age of pregnancy	Age (days)	
Case 1										

Table 4. Data registration case identification proposal.

Biological fresh samples collected should include abortion material, foetus, placenta, umbilical cord (**Figure 9**) and maternal blood samples but, at the local, photos must be taken and description of gross lesions must be done, as proposed in **Tables 5** and **6**.

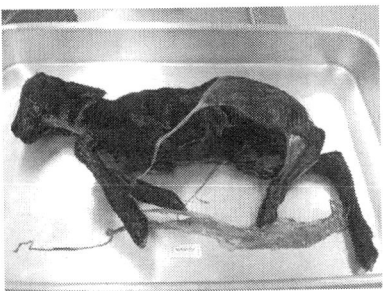

Figure 9. Complete abortion material collection, including foetus, placenta, umbilical cord of a stillborn lamb.

Arthrogryposis	Torticollis	Scoliosis	Kyphosis	Thickness of cranial bones	Flattened chest	Prognathism	Brachygnathia
Case 1							

Table 5. Musculoskeletal malformations registration.

Microcephaly	Cerebellar hypoplasia	Spinal cord hypoplasia	Lissencephaly	Hydranencephaly	Muscle atrophy	Other lesions	No gross lesions
Case 1							

Table 6. CNS malformations registration.

However, the shipment of biological fresh samples represents one of the greatest challenges in the diagnosis of SVB, once abortion is very common and the abortion products are found in the field, already in an advanced state of putrefaction and autolysis (**Figures 8** and **9**).

2. The vector of Schmallenberg virus in Portugal: lessons learned from the past and applications to the future

Blue tongue virus and African horse sickness virus (AHSV) are arboviruses that have circulated in Portugal in the past [11]. Both BTV and AHSV are double-stranded RNA viruses from the family Reoviridae that cause infectious, non-contagious illness, included in List A diseases by the Office International des Epizooties. BTV affects all species of ruminants [12], whereas

AHSV affects equines and occasionally dogs [10]. These arboviruses are transmitted by the bites of vector species of *Culicoides* [13]. Thus, so as with Schmallenberg, the incidence and geographical distribution of BTV and AHSV are associated to the distribution and abundance of *Culicoides*. *Culicoides imicola* constitutes the only field vector of AHSV while being the main vector of BTV in Europe and Africa [11].

Both BTV and AHSV have sporadically emerged into the southern European countries of the Mediterranean basin with the largest epidemic of BTV occurring between 1998 and 2002, and affecting Bulgaria, Greece, Turkey, Italy, Macedonia, Yugoslavia, Spain, France, Montenegro, Serbia and Bosnia and Herzegovina [14, 15]. Interestingly, BTV northern spread has shown novel territories of *C. imicola* expansion, which is believed to have been influenced by global warming [16].

Given the epizootic features of BTV, there was the constant need to record the distribution of *C. imicola* and to identify whether other potential vector species of the *Culicoides* genus are sufficiently distributed and in sufficient numbers to act as vectors for sustained arbovirus transmission, and also to map areas of higher risk for endemicity of BTV and ASHV due to the constant presence of adult *Culicoides* vectors [11]. These goals have for the past years been achieved by vector surveillance systems across Mediterranean Europe and bordering countries, thus producing detailed predictive risk maps of *Culicoides*-borne disease.

Discussing this topic shows the need to highlight two reports of *Culicoides* vector surveillance carried out in Portugal [11, 17], which mostly cover all territories and provide detailed information on the temporal distribution of *Culicoides* species in Portugal from 2000 to 2010, as independent entomological surveys.

Both studies have assumed similar sampling schemes, and divided mainland Portugal into 45 quadrats (or geographical units) each 50 km × 50 km so as to cover all territories in detail (**Figure 10**) and performed similar trapping strategies.

Capela et al. [11] sampled a total of 87 sites (including at least two livestock holdings or farms) within almost all geographical units. The authors took into account for variations in environmental conditions between sampling years, randomly dividing into two equal groups and sampling the first in 2000 and the second in 2001. Farms were included in the study if fulfilling the following criteria: located at least 10 km apart and 2.5 km from the coast, contained a minimum of five large livestock animals and did not use insecticides. Trapping was performed using Onderstepoort-type black light traps [18, 19] with 8-W UV light bulbs and downdraught suction, set on each night between 1 h before sunset to approximately 08.00 h the following morning. Traps were set outside but within 25 m of livestock. Ribeiro et al. [17] sampled a total of 212 sites within all geographical units between 2005 and 2010. Farms were included in the study if fulfilling the following criteria: located at a minimum distance of 10 km from other sampled holdings and at least 2.5 km from the coast, and contain a minimum of five horses or ruminants (preferably cattle). Recruited farms were also not permitted to enforce insecticide application for the duration of the survey. Trapping was performed using Center for Disease Control (CDC) miniature light traps (model 1212; John W. Hock, Gainesville, FL, USA) with a

4-W UV light and a suction fan, set from dusk to dawn. Traps were set outside but within 30 m from livestock.

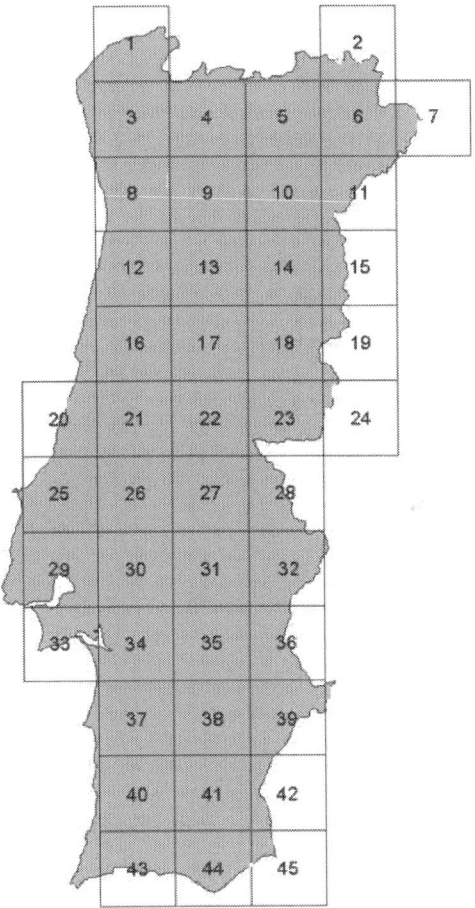

Figure 10. Sampling frames for *Culicoides* entomological surveys in Portugal since 2000 [11, 17].

2.1. Step one 2000–2001

During summer, 166 samples were collected containing 55,937 *Culicoides* spp. Individuals [11]. *Culicoides imicola* was the most frequently observed species, accounting for 66% of all individuals, followed by *C. obsoletus* (17.3%) and *C. pulicaris* (10.7%), and with *C. puncticollis* and other *Culicoides* complexes accounting for a very low proportion among all individuals. Despite being found at higher numbers, *C. imicola* was less prevalent across geographical units (found in 64%) than either *C. obsoletus* (found in 82%) or *C. pulicaris* (found in 93%). *Culicoides imicola* was significantly more prevalent in south Portugal (91% of southern geographical units) than north Portugal (42% of northern geographical units). The most northern site positive for *C. imicola* in this study was at 41°38.4' N. *Culicoides imicola* was collected until the maximum altitude of 850 m above sea level. *Culicoides imicola* appeared to be absent from the north-west corner of Portugal and along the north-west coast. On the contrary, *C. imicola* was found to be highly abundant in the central eastern Portugal. During winter, 22,883 individuals of *Culicoides* spp. were collected with *C. pulicaris* accounting for 47% of the total *Culicoides* spp. catch, followed by *C. obsoletus* (6%) and *C. imicola* (1%).

2.2. Step two 2005–2010

Of the total 5800 catches, 3632 contained *Culicoides* species [17]. *Culicoides imicola* was the most frequently observed species, accounting for 74.8% of the individuals, followed by *C. obsoletus* (7.7%). The central region of the country accounted for the highest catches of *C. imicola*. *Culicoides imicola* was found to be less prevalent than *C. obsoletus* and comparing the distribution data with the one reported in 2000–2001 [20], *C. imicola* was found in five more geographical units, mainly in the northern regions. *Culicoides imicola* prevalence (per geographical unit) was higher in both central and southern regions when compared to the north. The most northern site positive for *C. imicola* in this study was at 41°92' N. *Culicoides imicola* was collected until the maximum altitude of 1694 m above sea level. *Culicoides imicola* was found to be highly abundant in the central region of the country. The largest collections of *C. imicola* occurred during the summer months of July, August and September, and the lowest during the winter months of December, January and February.

2.3. Overall analysis 2000–2010

When combined, both studies provide robust evidence that *C. imicola* has been the most prevalent *Culicoides* species in Portugal for the decade between 2000 and 2010, followed by members of the *Obsoletus* group, clearly showing the sustained presence of Schmallenberg virus vectors across the territory [11, 17].

Both studies also provide strong support to the notion that *C. imicola* is more prevalent in the central and south of Portugal, while the *Obsoletus* group is more widespread throughout the territory. Preferences in vector distribution have been related to different climate and habitat particularities, which are markedly distinct between the north and the central/south regions in Portugal [21]. Mainland Portugal geography is clearly demarcated by both the Atlantic at the north and the Mediterranean at the south with a borderline set across the territory and defined by Tagus, dividing the north with its forests, valleys and mountains, and the south with its vast lowlands where typical Mediterranean vegetation grows [17]. Climate is also diverse with maritime features and sharp differences between seasons in the north, and dry hot climate in the south. Higher prevalence of *C. imicola* in the south has been associated to the vector preference for breeding in moist nutrient-rich soils with high exposure to sun, typical features of southern regions of Portugal [17], and a preference not observed for *Obsoletus* group [20].

Both reports also show that over the 10-year time frame of 2000–2010, *C. imicola* has been detected more to the north but also at higher altitudes (850 m vs 1645 m) supporting that the vector is adapting and spreading to newer territories. Nonetheless, the authors report that the low numbers found suggest that these locations may be of borderline suitability, and the specimens caught could potentially have been wind-borne from more suitable regions [17, 22]. In conclusion, combined entomological data from both Capela et al. [11] and Ribeiro et al. [17] increase the understanding of the ecology of *Culicoides* vectors and *Culicoides* activity in Portugal. They provide important data on vectors that are known to have a significant impact on ruminants, in particular and within the scope of this review, of interest to Schmallenberg virus epidemiology in Portugal and in the support to design strategies to prevent disease spread in Portugal.

Author details

Fernando Esteves[1,2], João Rodrigo Mesquita[1,2,3*], Cármen Nóbrega[1,2], Carla Santos[1,2], António Monteiro[1,2], Rita Cruz[1,2], Helena Vala[1,2,4] and Ana Cláudia Coelho[5]

*Address all correspondence to: jmesquita@esav.ipv.pt

1 Agrarian Superior School of Viseu, Polytechnic Institute of Viseu, Viseu, Portugal

2 Centre for the Study of Education, Technologies and Health (CI&DETS), Polytechnic Institute of Viseu, Viseu, Portugal

3 CIBIO/UP, Research Center in Biodiversity and Genetic Resources/University of Porto, Vairão, Portugal

4 Centre for the Research and Technology of Agro-Environmental and Biological Sciences (CITAB), Vila Real, Portugal

5 Department of Veterinary Sciences, University of Trás-os-Montes and Alto Douro, Vila Real, Portugal

References

[1] Herder V, Hansmann F, Wohlsein P, Peters M, Varela M, Palmarini M, Baumgärtner W. Immunophenotyping of inflammatory cells associated with Schmallenberg virus infection of the central nervous system of ruminants. PLoS One. 2013;8(5):e62939.

[2] Agerholm JS, Hewicker-Trautwein M, Peperkamp K, Windsor PA. Virus-induced congenital malformations in cattle. Acta Vet Scand. 2015;57:54.

[3]   Balseiro A, Royo LJ, Gómez Antona A, García Marín JF. First Confirmation of Schmallenberg Virus in Cattle in Spain: Tissue Distribution and Pathology. Transbound Emerg Dis. 2015, 62(5):e62–5. doi: 10.1111/tbed.12185.

[4]   Lievaart-Peterson K, Luttikholt S, Peperkamp K, Van den Brom R, Vellema P. Schmallenberg disease in sheep or goats: past, present and future. Vet Microbiol. 2015;181(1–2):147–53.

[5]   Peperkamp NH, Luttikholt SJ, Dijkman R, Vos JH, Junker K, Greijdanus S, Roumen MP, van Garderen E, Meertens N, van Maanen C, Lievaart K, van Wuyckhuise L, Wouda W. Ovine and bovine congenital abnormalities associated with intrauterine infection with Schmallenberg virus. Vet Pathol. 2015;52(6):1057–66. doi: 10.1177/0300985814560231 [Epub 2014 Nov 26].

[6]   van den Brom R, Luttikholt SJ, Lievaart-Peterson K, Peperkamp NH, Mars MH, van der Poel WH, Vellema P. Epizootic of ovine congenital malformations associated with Schmallenberg virus infection. Tijdschr Diergeneeskd. 2012;137(2):106–11.

[7]   Hahn K, Habierski A, Herder V, Wohlsein P, Peters M, Hansmann F, Baumgärtner W. Schmallenberg virus in central nervous system of ruminants. Emerg Infect Dis. 2013;19(1):154–155.

[8]   Varela M, Schnettler E, Caporale M, Murgia C, Barry G. Schmallenberg virus pathogenesis, tropism and interaction with the innate immune system of the host. PLOS Pathog. 2013;9(1):e1003133. doi: 10.1371/journal.ppat.1003133.

[9]   Herder V, Wohlsein P, Peters M, Hansman F, Baumgärtner W. Vet Pathol. 2012;49(4) 588–591.

[10] Mellor PS, Boorman J. The transmission and geographical spread of African horse sickness and bluetongue viruses. Ann Tropical Med Parasitol. 1995;89:1–15.

[11] Capela R, Purse BV, Pena I, Wittman EJ, Margarita Y, Capela M, Romão L, Mellor PS, Baylis M. Spatial distribution of Culicoides species in Portugal in relation to the transmission of African horse sickness and bluetongue viruses. Med Vet Entomol. 2003;17(2): 165–77.

[12] Taylor WP. The epidemiology of bluetongue. Rev Sci Tech Off Int Epizoot. 1986;5:351–356.

[13] Mellor PS, Boorman J, Baylis M. Culicoides biting midges, their role as arbovirus vectors. Ann Rev Entomol. 2000;45:307–340.

[14] Mellor PS, Wittmann EJ. Bluetongue virus in the Mediterranean basin, 1998–2001. Vet J. 2002;164:20–37.

[15] Baylis M. The re-emergence of bluetongue. Vet J. 2002;164:5–6.

[16] Wittmann EJ, Baylis M. Climate change, effects on Culicoides-transmitted viruses and implications for the UK. Vet J. 2000;160:107–117.

[17] Ribeiro R, Wilson AJ, Nunes T, Ramilo DW, Amador R, Madeira S, Baptista FM, Harrup LE, Lucientes J, Boinas F. Spatial and temporal distribution of *Culicoides* species in mainland Portugal (2005–2010). Results of the Portuguese Entomological Surveillance Programme. PLoS One. 2015;10(4):e0124019.

[18] Nevill CG, Watkins WM, Carter JY, Munafu CG, et al. Comparison of mosquito nets, proguanil hydrochloride, and placebo to prevent malaria. BMJ. 1988;297(6645):401–403.

[19] Venter GJ, Sweatman GK. Seasonal abundance and parity of *Culicoides* biting midges associated with livestock at Roma, Lesotho (Diptera: Ceratopogonidae). Onderstepoort J Vet Res. 1989;56(3):173–177.

[20] Scientific Opinion of the Panel on Animal Health and Welfare on a request from the European Commission (DGSANCO) on Bluetongue. The EFSA Journal (2008) 735, 1–70.

[21] Ramilo DW, Diaz S, Pereira da Fonseca I, Delécolle J- C, Wilson A, Meireles J, et al. First report of 13 species of *Culicoides* (Diptera: Ceratopogonidae) in mainland Portugal and azores by morphological and molecular characterization. PLoS One. 2012;7(4):e34896.

[22] García-Lastra R, Leginagoikoa I, Plazaola JM, Ocabo B, Aduriz G, Nunes T, et al. Bluetongue virus serotype 1 outbreak in the Basque country (Northern Spain) 2007–2008. Data Support a Primary Vector Windborne Transport. Gubbins S, editor. PLoS One. 2012;7(3):e34421.

Epidemiology of Non-Communicable Disease

The Epidemiological, Morphological, and Clinical Aspects of the Aberrant Right Subclavian Artery (Arteria Lusoria)

Michał Polguj, Ludomir Stefańczyk and
Mirosław Topol

Additional information is available at the end of the chapter

http://dx.doi.org/10.5772/64604

Abstract

The most common embryologic abnormality of the aortic arch is aberrant right subclavian artery (ARSA), known clinically as arteria lusoria (AL). This vessel travels to the right arm, crossing the middle line of the body and usually passing behind the esophagus. If the artery compresses the esophagus, it may produce a condition called dysphagia lusoria. Another commonly reported symptoms related to compression of adjacent structures by arteria lusoria were dyspnea, retrosternal pain, cough, and weight loss greater than 10 kg over a 6-month period. The chapter includes information describing demographic, clinical, and morphological characteristics of presence of arteria lusoria such as gender distribution, frequency in population, frequency of the most commonly reported symptoms related to compression of adjacent structures, coexistence with the most common vascular anomalies and diagnostic procedures. The presence of arteria lusoria together with the right nonrecurrent inferior laryngeal nerve (NRILN) is especially clinically important; during thyroid surgery, the right laryngeal nerve cannot be found at the lower pole of the thyroid, and it may be injured by the surgeon if it is not identified in the aberrant area or found lateral to the thyroid.

Keywords: aberrant right subclavian artery, arteria lusoria, anatomical variations, vessels, clinical symptoms

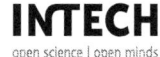

1. Introduction

The one of the most common embryologic vascular abnormalities of the aortic arch is an aberrant right subclavian artery (ARSA), known clinically as arteria lusoria (AL) [1].

In approximately 80% of individuals, three arteries arise from the arch of the aorta. From right to left, the brachiocephalic trunk arises (divided into the right common carotid artery and the right subclavian artery), followed by the left common carotid artery, and finally the left subclavian artery (**Figure 1**) [2].

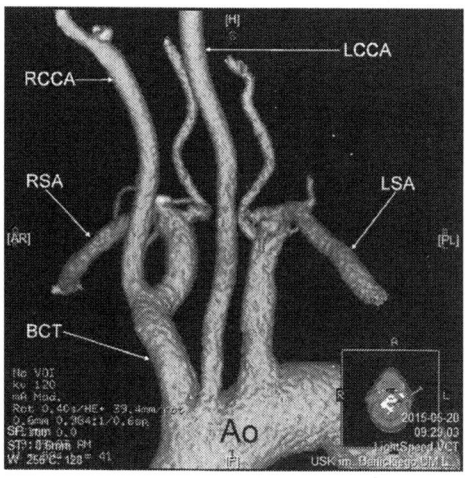

Figure 1. Three-dimensional computed tomography reconstruction of the arteries (CT-64-row MDCT scanner, Lightspeed VCT, GE, Waukesha, Wisconsin, USA). Ao—arch of the aorta, BCT—brachiocephalic trunk, LSA—left subclavian artery, LCCA—left common carotid artery, RCCA—right common carotid artery, RSA—right subclavian artery.

When an aberrant right subclavian artery (arteria lusoria) is present, the brachiocephalic trunk is absent and four arteries arise from the arch of the aorta: the right common carotid artery followed by the left common carotid artery, the left subclavian artery, and finally the right subclavian artery, with the most distal left-sided origin (**Figures 2–4**). This vessel, the aberrant right subclavian artery, travels to the right arm, crossing the middle line of the body and usually passing behind the esophagus (**Figure 3**) [3, 4]. If the artery compresses neighboring structures or organs, it may produce symptoms, the most common example being compression of the esophagus by the arteria lusoria, which results in a condition called dysphagia lusoria [4].

Although the first description of an aberrant right subclavian artery was provided in 1735 by Hunauld, the clinical entity was presented later [2]. In 1794, David Bayford, a physician from London, England, described a 33-year-old woman who succumbed to malnutrition after 20 years of progressive dysphagia [3]. At autopsy, Dr. Bayford noted esophageal compression by an abnormal right subclavian artery and suggested the term "dysphagia lusoria" to describe this syndrome. Hence, it is also known as Bayford–Autenrieth dysphagia [3]. Kommerell described its radiological findings in 1936 [4].

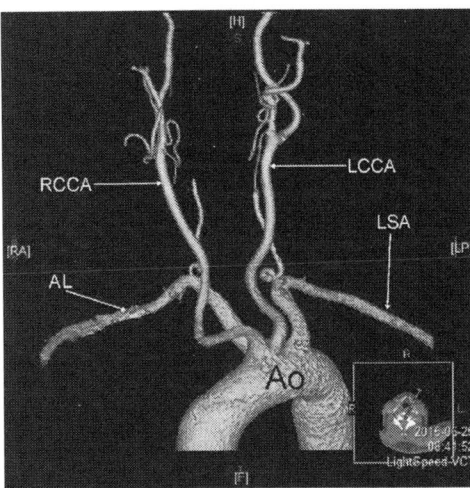

Figure 2. Three-dimensional computed tomography reconstruction of the arteries (CT-64-row MDCT scanner, Lightspeed VCT, GE, Waukesha, Wisconsin, USA). Ao—arch of the aorta, AL—arteria lusoria, LSA—left subclavian artery, LCCA—left common carotid artery, RCCA—right common carotid artery.

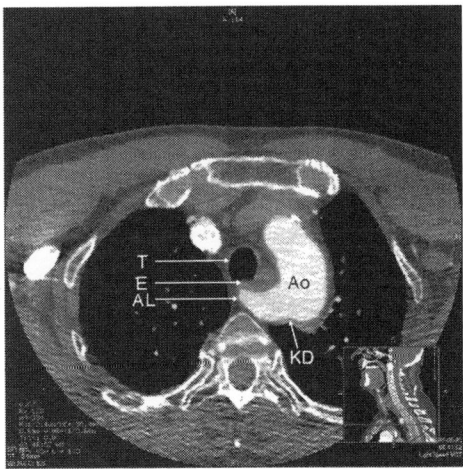

Figure 3. Computed tomography transverse scan on the level of arch of the aorta. Ao—arch of the aorta, AL—arteria lusoria, E—esophagus, KD—Kommerell's diverticulum, T—trachea.

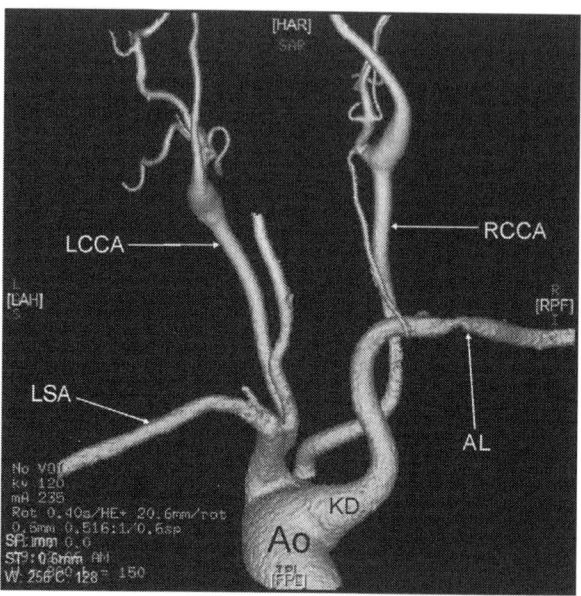

Figure 4. Three-dimensional computed tomography reconstruction of the arteries (CT-64-row MDCT scanner, Light-Speed VCT, GE, Waukesha, Wisconsin, USA). Ao—arch of the aorta, AL—arteria lusoria, KD—Kommerell's diverticulum, LSA—left subclavian artery, LCCA—left common carotid artery, RCCA—right common carotid artery.

2. Embryology

Arteria lusoria results from abnormal embryologic development of the aortic arch. In the normal situation, between the 4th and 5th weeks of embryonic life, blood leaves the heart by a common trunk called the "truncus arteriosus", which divides into two branches termed the ventral aortae. These branches are connected with the paired dorsal aortae by six aortic arches. The carotid system is formed by segments of the first three arches. The right fourth arch, a segment of the right ventral aorta, and a portion of the right dorsal aorta develop into the right subclavian artery. The left fourth arch persists as the adult aortic arch with the anlagen of the seventh dorsal intersegmental artery, and this forms the left subclavian artery. The fifth arches are both resorbed, and the sixth arches form the pulmonary artery and the ductus arteriosus [5, 6].

The aberrant origin of the right subclavian artery is caused by the involution of the right fourth vascular arch and proximal right dorsal aorta and the persistence of the seventh intersegmental artery originating from the proximal descending thoracic aorta, resulting in the arteria lusoria following an abnormal course [5, 6].

3. Epidemiological and demographic characteristics

The frequency of ARSA varies throughout the world. In Europe, depending on the country, it has been found in 0.11% (Great Britain) [7], 0.16% (Greece) [8], 0.3% (France) [9], or 0.36% (the Netherlands) [10] of the population. Studies have also been performed on other continents: Asia, 0.1–0.2% of cases (respectively: China and Japan) [11, 12]; North America, 0.5% of cases (United State) [13]; or Australia and Oceania, 0.8% of cases (New Zealand) [14] (**Table 1**). However, its detection arguably depends primarily on the sensitivity of the diagnostic procedures employed, for example, cadaveric or CT versus chest X-ray examination.

AL (%)	Country	Type of investigation	N/(total)	Researcher
0.1	China	Angiography	3/3000	Nie et al. [11]
0.11	Great Britain	Gastroscopy	1/920	Kelly [7]
0.16	Greece	Angiography	1/622	Natsis et al. [8]
0.2	Japan	Autopsy	1/516	Saito et al. [12]
0.3	France	coronarography	11/3730	Abhaichand et al. [9]
0.36	The Netherlands	Endoesophageal ultrasonography	12/3334	De Luca et al. [10]
0.5	USA	Computed tomography	36/7174	Haesemeyer and Gavant [13]
0.8	New Zealand	Autopsy	19/2291	Cainey [14]

AL—arteria lusoria.

Table 1. Frequency of aberrant right subclavian artery (arteria lusoria) in different populations.

The gender distribution of the aberrant right subclavian artery was found to be similar: 55.3% females versus 44.7% males [15].

4. Clinical characteristics

An aberrant right subclavian artery is usually asymptomatic, while about 8–10% of adult patients develop symptoms [16]. The anomaly does not cause symptoms in most patients and can be discovered incidentally during life or found at autopsy [17, 18].

When present, symptoms usually occur at the two extremes of life [19]. In children, respiratory symptoms are prevalent, mainly dyspnea or chronic coughing. They can also present with repetitive respiratory infections. Infant patients may demonstrate an increased frequency of pulmonary infections, which is thought to be due to absence of tracheal rigidity in combination with dysphagia and aspiration [19, 20]. As noted above, a rare cause of dysphagia observed in adults is compression of the esophagus by an abnormal course of the aberrant right subclavian artery, which is classically termed "dysphagia lusoria" [3].

Although dysphagia may be the most frequent symptom demonstrated by adults, children demonstrate a different respiratory symptomatology attributed to lack of the tracheal rigidity associated with dysphagia and false routes [21]. In addition, the arteria lusoria can also be revealed by the extension of aortic dissection or by peripheral arterial embolism.

A meta-analysis by Polguj et al. found the most commonly reported symptoms related to compression of adjacent structures by an aberrant right subclavian artery to be dysphagia (71.2%), dyspnea (18.7%), retrosternal pain (17.0%), cough (7.6%), and weight loss greater than 10 kg over a six-month period (5.9%) [15]. Among the less common symptoms, stomachache, back pain, and numbness of the right upper limb were reported. The mean age of the onset of symptoms was 49.9 ± 19.4 years for the whole group (data shown as mean ± standard deviation). However, the mean age according to gender was 44.9 ± 18.1 years for males and 54.0 ± 19.6 years for females. This difference was statistically significant [15].

Dysphagia also frequently occurs in elderly patients, for which four mechanisms have been proposed: increased rigidity of the trachea leading to easy compression of esophagus, aneurysm formation, presence of Kommerell's diverticulum, elongation of the aorta, the coexistence of an aberrant artery with a truncus bicaroticus, or a close origin of common carotid arteries from the arch of the aorta [22–25].

To the angiographer who uses the right axillary, brachial or radial approach to the ascending thoracic aorta, the arteria lusoria is also a clinically important element. The presence of an ARSA is suspected in cases in which catheterization of the ascending aorta proves difficult. Using the right radial approach, access to the ascending aorta is usually easy [11]. Previous studies indicate that only 60% of such cases were successfully performed by transradial approach in the setting of AL [26]. This variant makes the right transradial route difficult to approach the ascending aorta, as it requires the catheter to curve back to reach the aortic root [26, 27]. However, the repeated entry of the guide wire from the right subclavian artery to the descending aorta rather than the ascending aorta should indicate this possibility. Thus, angiography can prove to be very challenging in the presence of an arteria lusoria [11, 26, 27].

Finally, the inferior right recurrent laryngeal nerve is an asymptomatic variation anomaly, which can be an important obstacle and be seriously damaged during cervicotomy, thyroid, and parathyroid surgery. In such cases, the inferior right recurrent laryngeal nerve is a classic risk and must be eliminated by location and routine dissection of the nerve [28–30]. This is of particular importance when the diagnosis concerns an asymptomatic neural anomaly discovered by dissection or a vascular anomaly whose symptoms are very variable [30].

5. Morphological characteristics

The literature presents two main classifications of the aberrant right subclavian artery. According to Neuhauser's threefold classification, the first type of arteria lusoria crosses the posterior wall of the esophagus, and this is observed in more than 80% of the cases. In the second type, this artery passes between the trachea and the esophagus (15% of the cases), and in the third type, it crosses the midline of the body ahead of the trachea (in 5% of the cases) [23].

In contrast, the Adachi and Williams classification recognizes four basic morphological types. Type I/G is characterized by an aberrant right subclavian artery arising from the arch of the aorta as the final branch. Type II/CG is similar to the first type, but an additional left vertebral artery arises from the arch of the aorta. In type III/H, three arteries arise from the arch of the aorta: as the first common trunk of the common carotid arteries (truncus bicaroticus), as the left subclavian artery, and as the last aberrant right subclavian artery. In type IV/N, the aberrant left subclavian artery arises from the right-sided arch of the aorta as the final branch [31].

The most common vascular anomalies coexisting with an aberrant right subclavian artery (arteria lusoria) were found to be truncus bicaroticus (19–29%), Kommerell's diverticulum (15–60%), aneurysm (just after the origin of arteria lusoria) (13%), and right-sided aortic arch (9%) [15]. Klinkhamer regards truncus bicaroticus is a precondition for tracheal–esophageal compression and the development of clinical symptoms. Under these circumstances, the truncus bicaroticus holds the trachea from the front, and the aberrant right subclavian artery compresses the esophagus from behind [22].

In 1936, Kommerell published the first radiological findings of the route of the aortic arch as an aortic diverticulum (Kommerell's diverticulum), which was identified as being located at the origin of an aberrant subclavian artery [4] (**Figure 3** and **4**). Kommerell's diverticulum is usually found incidentally on a chest roentgenogram and is often misdiagnosed as a mediastinal tumor [29]. Kommerell's diverticulum is a normal broadening of the proximal origin of the aberrant right subclavian artery from the aortic arch and is most frequently present in patients with a right aortic arch and an aberrant left subclavian artery [32]. However, Kommerell's diverticulum is not analogous with an aneurysm: The primary indication for surgical repair of Kommerell's diverticulum is a diameter larger than 50 mm and the presence of clinical symptoms.

The identification of arteria lusoria should alert the radiologist and surgeon that a nonrecurrent inferior laryngeal nerve (NRILN) is present and that an anticipating surgical technique should be performed to reduce the risk of neural injury. Due to its anatomical position, an NRILN is not only at risk of being damaged during thyroidectomy, but also during such other surgical procedures as neck dissection, parathyroidectomy, and carotid endarterectomy [30, 33].

6. Diagnosis

The diagnosis of arteria lusoria was reported only on anatomical dissection until 1936, when Burckhard Kommerell described the clinical diagnosis of an aberrant right subclavian artery that originated from an aortic diverticulum, later known as Kommerell's diverticulum, in a 65-year-old man who was believed to have stomach cancer [4]. In 1946, Gross was the first to report the surgical treatment of dysphagia lusoria, in a four-month-old infant [34].

The diagnostic modalities available to visualize an arteria lusoria include barium esophago-gram, computed tomography (CT), magnetic resonance imaging (MRI), digital subtraction angiography (DSA), endoscopy and endoscopic ultrasound. New advances in CT technology allow even small vascular structures to be visualized in detail. Multidetector computed tomography (MDCTA) is now an established diagnostic test in the evaluation of many vascular diseases [35–39].

Barium contrast examination of the esophagus shows a characteristic, extrinsic, smooth diagonal impression at the level of the third and fourth dorsal vertebra. Lateral or oblique views show the extrinsic impression to be posterior, and in case of arteria lusoria, just above the level of the aortic arch. As dysphagia occurs frequently with ingestion of solid foods, including a barium soaked bread bolus may improve localization of the defect [35].

Digital subtraction angiography gives valuable information regarding AL. It is an invasive procedure and, in contrast to MDCT, has the disadvantage in showing extravascular structures such as the esophagus. It has also been shown that the effective radiation doses in MDCT angiography studies are moderate and even lower than those associated with DSA in a comparable patient group.

CT or MRI (magnetic resonance imaging) angiography has replaced conventional angiog-raphy and is the gold standard for the diagnosis. It not only confirms the diagnosis but also helps to exclude aneurysm of the aorta or other associated anomalies and to plan the operation [36–39].

MRI has the advantage of being a noninvasive procedure and the patient is spared the potential risk of intravenous contrast agents. MRI is not as useful as MDCT due to the generation of respiratory and cardiac motion artifacts. Also it is not a preferred method due to its cost and prolonged scan time. Although MR angiography may reveal the pres-ence of a vascular anomaly, the information regarding nonvascular mediastinal structures is insufficient [36–39].

Endoscopy may reveal pulsatile, shelf-like extrinsic compression in the posterior wall of the esophagus, with intact mucosa. Such an area of narrowing is usually located between 20 and 24 cm from the mouth [7].

Endoscopic ultrasound (EUS) can identify an arteria lusoria, as it lies close to the esophagus. EUS is regarded as the most accurate test for the evaluation of the esophageal wall and the surrounding structures, with the incorporation of Doppler technology in modern echoendo-scopes allowing particularly accurate examination of adjacent vessels [10].

The combination of MDCT with 3D volume rendering images provides further advantages. These allow not only the depiction of the thoracic vascular anomalies but also more accurate assessment of the diameter, angle, and compressed area of the esophagus and the relationship between the AL with the esophagus and other mediastinal structures. In addition, MDCT is a noninvasive procedure, unlike DSA, and offers easier application and a shorter time require-ment than DSA or MRA [36–39].

7. Conclusion

A familiarity with the anatomy of the some types of vascular anomalies is necessary for clinicians involved in many medical areas. Compression of adjacent structures by an arteria lusoria needs to be differentiated from other conditions presenting symptoms such as dysphagia, dyspnea, retrosternal pain, cough, and weight loss. The knowledge presented in this chapter will allow the best healthcare to be provided for patients.

Author details

Michał Polguj[1*], Ludomir Stefańczyk[2] and Mirosław Topol[3]

*Address all correspondence to: michal.polguj@umed.lodz.pl

1 Department of Angiology, Medical University of Łódź, Łódź, Poland

2 Department of Radiology, Medical University of Łódź, Łódź, Poland

3 Department of Normal and Clinical Anatomy, Medical University of Łódź, Łódź, Poland

References

[1] Molz G, Burri B. Aberrant subclavian artery (arteria lusoria): sex differences in the prevalence of various forms of the malformation. Evaluation of 1378 observations. Virchows Arch A Pathol Anat Histol. 1978, 380(4): 303–15

[2] Hunauld PM. Examen de quelques parties d'un singe. Hist Acad Roy Sci. 1735;2:516–23.

[3] Bayford D. An account of a singular case of obstructed deglutition. Mem M Society London. 1794, 2, 275–86.

[4] Kommerell B. Verlagerung des Osophagus durch eine abnorm verlaufende Arteria subclavia dextra (arteria lusoria). Fortschr Geb Roentgenstrahlen. 1936, 54: 590–95.

[5] Kopp R, Wizgall J, Kreuzer E, Meimarakis G, Weidenhagen R, Kiiknl A, Conrad C, Jauch KW, Lauterjun L. Surgical and endovascular treatment of symptomatic aberrant right subclavian artery (arteria lusoria). Vascular. 2007, 15: 84–91.

[6] Inami T, Seino Y, Mizuno K. Unique case of giant Kommerell diverticulum with aberrant left subclavian artery arising from the left aortic arch associated with situs inversus. Int J Cardiol. 2013, 163(3): e47–48.

[7] Kelly MD. Endoscopy and the aberrant right subclavian artery. Am Surg. 2007, 73(12): 1259–61.

[8]   Natsis KI, Tsitouridis IA, Didagelos MV, Fillipidis AA, Vlasis KG, Tsikaras PD. Anatomical variations in the branches of the human aortic arch in 633 angiographies: clinical significance and literature review. Surg Radiol Anat. 2009, 31(5): 319–23.

[9]   Abhaichand RK, Louvard Y, Gobeil JF, Loubeyre C, Lefèvre T, Morice MC. The problem of arteria lusoria in right transradial coronary angiography and angioplasty. Catheter Cardiovasc Interv. 2001, 54(2): 196–01.

[10] De Luca L, Bergman JJ, Tytgat GN, Fockens P. EUS imaging of the arteria lusoria: case series and review. Gastrointest Endosc. 2000, 52(5): 670–73.

[11] Nie B, Zhou YJ, Li GZ, Shi DM, Wang JL. Clinical study of arterial anatomic variations for transradial coronary procedure in Chinese population. Chin Med J (Engl) 2009, 122(18): 2097–02.

[12] Saito T, Tamatsukuri Y, Hitosugi T, Miyakawa K, Shimizu T, Oi Y, Yoshimoto M, Yamamoto Y, Spanel-Browski K, Steinke H. Three cases of retroesophageal right subclavian artery. J Nippon Med Sch. 2005, 72(6): 375–82.

[13] Haesemeyer SW, Gavant ML. Imaging of acute traumatic aortic tear in patients with an aberrant right subclavian artery. AJR Am J Roentgenol. 1999, 172(1): 117–20.

[14] Cainey J. Tortuosity of the cervical segment of the internal carotid artery. J Anat. 1924, 59(1): 87–96.

[15] Polguj M, Chrzanowski Ł, Kasprzak J, Stefanczyk L, Topol M, Majos A. The aberrant right subclavian artery (arteria lusoria) — the morphological and clinical aspects of the one of the most important variations: a systematic study of 141 reports. Sci World J. 2014;2014:292734.

[16] Delap TG, Jones SE, Johnson DR. Aneurysm of an aberrant right subclavian artery presenting as dysphagia lusoria. Ann Otol Rhinol Laryngol. 2000, 109(2): 231–34.

[17] Adachi B. Das Arteriensystem der Japener. Kenkyusha Press, Tokyo, Japan, 1928.

[18] Janssen M, Baggen MGA, Veen HF, Smout AJ, Bekkers JA, Jonkman JG, Ouwendijk RJ. Dysphagia lusoria: clinical aspects, manometric findings, diagnosis and therapy. Am J Gastroenterol. 2000, 96: 1411–16.

[19] Puri SK, Ghuman S, Narang P, Sharma A, Singh S. CT and MR angiography in dysphagia lusoria in adults. Ind J Radiol Imag. 2005, 15(4): 497–01.

[20] Van Son JA, Julsrud PR, Hagler DJ, Sim EK, Pairolero PC, Puga FJ, Schaff HV, Danielson GK. Surgical treatment of vascular rings: the Mayo Clinic experience. Mayo Clin Proc. 1993, 68: 1056–63.

[21] McNally PR, Rak KM. Dysphagia lusoria caused by persistent right aortic arch with aberrant left subclavian artery and diverticulum of kommerell. Dig Dis Sci. 1992, 37: 144–49.

[22] Klinkhamer AC. Aberrant right subclavian artery: clinical and roentgenologic aspects. Am J Roentgenol Radium Ther Nucl Med. 1966, 97: 438–46.

[23] Levitt B, Richter JE. Dysphagia lusoria: a comprehensive review. Dis Esophagus. 2007, 20: 455–60.

[24] Van Son JA, Mierzwa M, Mohr FM. Resection of atherosclerotic aneurysm at origin of aberrant right subclavian artery. Eur J Cardiovasc Surg. 1999, 16: 576–79.

[25] Ulger Z, Ozyurek AR, Levent E, Gurses D, Parlar A. Arteria lusoria as cause of dysphagia. Acta Cardiol. 2004, 59(4): 445–47.

[26] Valsecchi O, Vassileva A, Musumeci G, Rossini R, Tespili M, Guagliumi G, Mihalcsik L, Gavazzi A, Ferrazzi P. Failure of transradial approach during coronary interventions: anatomic considerations. Catheter Cardiovasc Interv. 2006, 67: 870–78.

[27] Huang IL, Hwang HR, Li SC, Chen CK, Liu CP, Wu MT. Dissection of arteria lusoria by transradial coronary catheterization: a rare complication evaluated by multidetector CT. J Chin Med Assoc. 2009, 72(7):379–81.

[28] Nakatani T, Tanaka S, Mizukami S, Okamoto K, Shiraishi Y, Nakamura T. Retroeso-phageal right subclavian artery originating from the aortic arch distal and dorsal to the left subclavian artery. Ann Anat. 1996, 178(3): 269–71.

[29] Epstein DA, Debord JR. Abnormalities associated with aberrant right subclavian arteries-a case report. Vasc Endovascular Surg. 2002, 36(4): 297–03.

[30] Avisse C, Marcus C, Delattre JF, Marcus C, Cailliez-Tomasi JP, Palot JP, Ladam-Marcus V, Menanteau B, Flament JB. Right nonrecurrent inferior laryngeal nerve and arteria lusoria: the diagnostic and therapeutic implications of an anatomic anomaly. Review of 17 cases. Surg Radiol Anat. 1998, 20(3):227–32.

[31] Williams GD, Aff HM, Schmeckebier M, Edmonds HW, Grand EG. Variations in the arrangement of the branches arising from the aortic arch in the American whites and Negroes. Anat Rec. 1932, 54: 247–51.

[32] Hartyanszky IL, Lozsadi K, Marcsek P, Huttl T, Sapi E, Kovacs AB. Congenital vascular rings: surgical management of 111 cases. Eur J Cardiothorac Surg. 1989, 3(3): 250–54.

[33] Devèze A, Sebag F, Hubbard J, Jaunay M, Maweja S, Henry JF. Identification of patients with a non-recurrent inferior laryngeal nerve by duplex ultrasound of the brachioce-phalic artery. Surg Radiol Anat. 2003, 25(3–4):263–9

[34] Gross RE. Surgical treatment for dysphagia lusoria. Ann Surg. 1946, 124:532–34.

[35] Branscom JJ, Austin JH. Aberrant right subclavian artery. Findings seen on plain chest roentgenograms. Am J Roentgenol Radium Ther Nucl Med. 1973, 119(3): 539–42.

[36] Alper F, Akgun M, Kantarci M, Eroglu A, Ceyhan E, Onbas O, Duran C, Okur A. Demonstration of vascular abnormalities compressing esophagus by MDCT: Special focus on dysphagia lusoria. Eur J Radiol. 2006, 59(1):82–7.

[37] Godlewski J, Widawski T, Michalak M, Kmieć Z Aneurysm of the aberrant right subclavian artery – a case report Pol J Radiol, 2010, 75(4): 47–50

[38] Chen X, Qu YJ, Peng ZY, Lu JG, Ma XJ. Diagnosis of congenital aortic arch anomalies in chinese children by multi-detector computed tomography angiography. J Huazhong Univ Sci Technolog Med Sci. 2013, 33(3): 447–51.

[39] Yang M, Mo XM, Jin JY, Wu M, Liu B, Liu ZY, Gao XC, Tang WW, Teng GJ. Diagnostic value of 64 multislice CT in typing of congenital aortic anomaly in neonates and infants. 2010, 90(31): 2167–71.

Factors Associated with Survival to Discharge of Newborns in a Middle-Income Country

Daynia Elizabeth Ballot and Tobias Chirwa

Additional information is available at the end of the chapter

http://dx.doi.org/10.5772/64306

Abstract

Clinical and mortality audit is an essential part of quality improvement in health care; information obtained in this process is used to develop targeted interventions to improve outcome. This study aimed to determine predictors of short-term survival in neonates. An existing neonatal database was reviewed. A total of 5018 neonates > 400 g admitted to a tertiary hospital (Johannesburg South Africa) between 1 January 2013 and 31 December 2015 were analysed. Mean birth weight was 2148 g (standard deviation [SD]: 972) and mean gestational age was 34.2 weeks (SD: 4.8). Overall survival was 85.6% (4294/5018). The most common causes of death were prematurity (46.2%), hypoxia (19.5%) and infection (17.2). The strongest predictors of survival were birth weight (OR 1.0; 95% confidence intervals (CI): 1.0–1.01) and gestational age (OR = 1.1, 95% CI: 1.05–1.17). Other predictors of survival included metabolic acidosis (OR = 0.14, 95% CI: 0.09–0.20), hyperglycemia (OR = 0.31, 95% CI: 0.23–0.41), mechanical ventilation (OR = 0.35, 95% CI: 0.28–0.46), major birth defect (OR = 0.12, 95% CI: 0.08–0.18), resuscitation at birth (OR = 0.39, 95% CI: 0.31–0.49) and Caesarean section (OR = 1.8, 95% CI: 1.44–2.25). In conclusion, resources need to be focused on improved care of VLBW infants.

Keywords: neonatal mortality, clinical audit, very low birth weight, premature infants

1. Introduction

The fourth Millennium Development Goal (MDG) was a two-third reduction in the mortality of children under the age of 5 years, which sub-Sahara African countries (including South Africa) failed to achieve this [1]. In 2015, 1 million children died within the first day of life, a further million in the first week of life and yet another 2.8 million in the first 28 days of life –

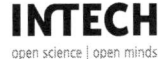

4.8 million of the almost 6 million children under the age of five years who died in 2015, died within the neonatal period [1]. Concentrating resources on newborns is therefore essential to further reduce childhood mortality.

The causes of neonatal mortality vary considerably among different units and different countries. The United Nations MDG 2015 report [1] states that "better data are needed for the post-2015 development agenda" and "real-time data are needed" to guide policy makers. Most data have a time lag of between 2 and 3 years before the policies are implemented. The MDGs formed the foundation of the so-called Sustainable Development Goals (SDG) [2]. The SDGs are less specific than the MDGs, but include health targets, one of which is to reduce both neonatal mortality and mortality of children under the age of 5 years.

Regular audits of neonatal mortality are required to identify the causes of death so that proper interventions can be implemented to reduce neonatal deaths. It is essential to have local data to address local health issues; transposing mortality data from another country will not necessarily solve local problems. This is particularly true when using data from a high-income country to address problems experienced in low- to middle-income countries (LMICS). A recent review of the mortality rates in neonatal intensive care units showed that the rate varied considerably between different countries [3]; the mortality rate was generally high, but greater in developing than developed countries. Issues such as the lack of antenatal care and inadequate health facilities are the causes of neonatal mortality in LMICS. A recent review from The Gambia [4] showed a high neonatal mortality rate – 35% of admitted neonates died. The important causes of neonatal death included lack of antenatal care, birth weight below 1500 g, hypothermia at birth, and delivery outside a teaching hospital.

Previous studies done in very low birth weight (VLBW) neonates – birth weight below 1500 g – at Charlotte Maxeke Johannesburg Academic Hospital (CMJAH) have shown that birth weight was the most significant predictor of survival [5, 6]. Resuscitation at birth, the use of nasal continuous positive airways pressure (NCPAP) and the mode of delivery were also important factors affecting survival. Survival of extremely low birth weight (ELBW) neonates was particularly low at CMJAH [7]. The provision of NCPAP to this category of neonates more than doubled their survival to discharge [6].

2. Determinants of neonatal survival at a tertiary hospital in Johannesburg, South Africa

Although VLBW mortality at CMJAH has been studied, the overall neonatal survival has not been audited. The aim of this study is to review neonatal survival at CMJAH and to determine important modifiable factors to inform protocols and budgeting for neonatal care. The objectives of this study were to:

- Describe the patient population with regard to demographic information, clinical characteristics, and outcome at discharge.

- Determine the survival rate for different birth weight categories.

- Establish factors associated with neonatal survival.

2.1. Subjects and methods

The study was conducted in the neonatal unit of a tertiary academic hospital (CMJAH) in Johannesburg, South Africa. All neonates admitted within 48 h of birth, between 1 January 2013 and 31 December 2015, were included in the study. Neonates with a birth weight below 400 g and those with important missing data, particularly birth weight, gestational age, and outcome at discharge were excluded.

2.2. Study design

This was a secondary analysis of an existing neonatal database. Data were collected upon discharge for each neonate admitted to the CMJAH neonatal unit and entered on to a database. The database was managed using Research Electronic Data Capture (REDCAP) [8] hosted by the University of the Witwatersrand. The information collected included demographic details, maternal information, delivery room data, clinical information, and outcome at discharge. Data from VLBW neonates was contributed to the Vermont Oxford Network (VON) (www.vtoxford.org), a multinational neonatal collaboration. A paper computer summary form was completed for each patient, using the patient file. Data were checked against the patient file and then entered on to the database. The information on the database was then checked against the paper form. Any discrepancies noted were verified against the patient files. Definitions and codes for congenital defects or surgical procedures were obtained from the VON.

Neonates were classified by weight using standard definitions—term large for gestational age (TLGA) neonates weighed above 4000 g at birth, term appropriate for gestational age (TAGA) infants weighed between 2500 and 3999 g at birth, low birth weight (LBW) neonates had a birth weight less than 2500 g, very low birth weight (VLBW) included those weighing less than 1500 g at birth and extremely low birth weight (ELBW) less than 1000 g at birth. Term was considered to be a gestation age between 37 and 42 weeks, preterm below 37 weeks, and post-term to be above 42 weeks.

The unit participated in a national perinatal mortality audit – the perinatal problem identification programme (PPIP)(www.ppip.co.za). The broad causes of neonatal death were categorized using standard PPIP definitions.

2.2.1. Neonatal unit

The neonatal unit was situated in large tertiary academic hospital in a metropolitan setting. Neonatal facilities included a transitional nursery in labour ward, a shared paediatric/neonatal intensive care unit (PNICU) with 15 ventilator beds, a neonatal high care unit with 40 beds, low-care facility with 25 beds, and nine kangaroo mother-care (KMC) beds. Nasal continuous positive airways pressure (NCPAP) and therapeutic hypothermia for perinatal asphyxia were provided in high care. The neonatal unit was staffed by neonatologists, registrars, and house staff. There were various paediatric sub-specialities in the hospital including nephrology, neurology, cardiology, endocrinology, and infectious diseases. There was a large paediatric surgery service and paediatric surgical neonates were admitted to the neonatal unit and jointly managed with the neonatal staff.

Neonates who were observed in the transitional unit and then discharged to their mothers were not included in the study. Neonates who died in the delivery room and transitional nursery were considered to be admissions and were included in the study. Owing to resource constraints, there were insufficient ventilator beds for the number of neonates requiring ventilation. The PNICU functioned essentially as a ventilator unit; high-care observation was not possible due to limited facilities. The neonatal unit had a policy of rationing care based on birth weight—babies weighing below 750 g at birth would not be offered surfactant or NCPAP, but only given supplemental oxygen, intravenous fluids, and antibiotics; babies weighing between 750 and 900 g would be given surfactant and NCPAP, but would not be provided with mechanical ventilation if required. All neonates with respiratory distress syndrome were initially managed with NCPAP and early rescue surfactant; those who failed would be transferred to the PNICU for mechanical ventilation. The use of NCPAP at CMJAH has recently been reviewed [9].

2.2.2. Statistical analysis

Data were exported to IBM SPSS version 22 for the purpose of analysis. The standard statistical methods were used to describe the data—continuous variables were described using measures of central tendency and dispersion, mean and standard deviation (SD), or median and interquartile range (IQR) as appropriate. Categorical variables were described using frequency and percentages.

The primary endpoint was whether a neonate survived to hospital discharge. Univariate analysis was done considering different maternal, demographic, and clinical variables as independent factors of survival. Differences in outcome for continuous variables were compared using unpaired t-tests or Mann Whitney U-test as appropriate. Associations of outcome with categorical variables were investigated using Chi-squared test. A factor with a p-value of 0.05 was considered statistically significant. Variables with a p-value <0.1 on the univariate analysis were entered into a multiple logistic regression model considering whether a child survived to discharge as the outcome variable. Factors associated with neonatal mortality were determined separately for VLBW and bigger babies.

The possible sources of bias were identified and excluded from the analysis. Conditions which were only present in neonates who were survivors and approaching discharge were identified and excluded from the analysis of deaths. These conditions included supplementary oxygen at 28 days, home oxygen and steroids for chronic lung disease. Maternal and delivery room conditions were compared between those neonates who died in the delivery room and those who died in the neonatal ward.

2.3. Ethics

Data were de-identified and the key to patient details was kept separately and only known to the principal investigator. Ethical clearance for the study was obtained from the Human Research Ethics Committee of the University of the Witwatersrand. Permission to conduct the study was obtained from the Chief Executive Officer of CMJAH. One of the authors was the gatekeeper of the neonatal database; additional permission to access the database was not required.

3. Results

The database was accessed on 20 February 2016, and there were 5695 neonatal records on the database; 5386 records were for neonates born within the study period. There were 26 records with missing outcome data, four babies who had a birth weight below 400 g and 338 neonates who were admitted to the unit after 48 h. Thus, 5018 records were included in the review. The mean birth weight was 2148 g (SD 972) and the mean gestational age was 34.2 weeks (SD 4.8). The mean duration of stay was 13.75 days (SD 18.0).

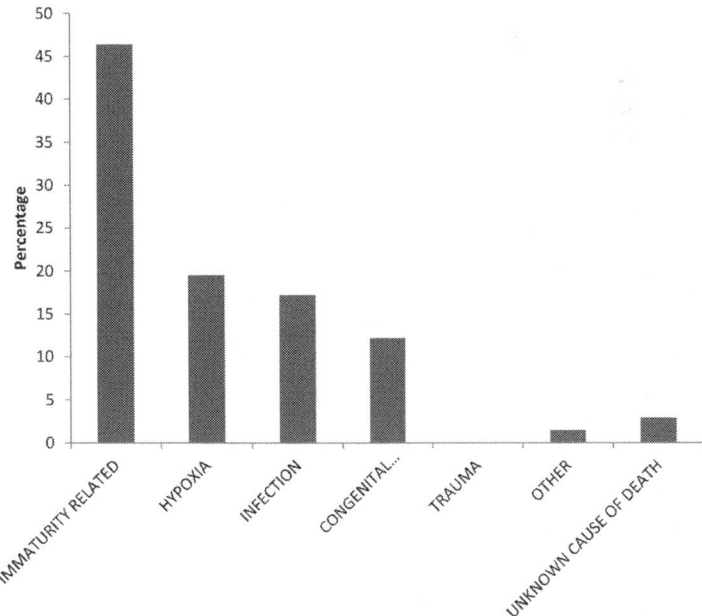

Figure 1. Causes of neonatal deaths in Johannesburg, South Africa, between 01 January 2013 and 31 December 2015.

There were 724 deaths, giving an overall mortality rate of 14.4%, alternatively expressed as a percentage surviving to discharge of 85.6. Seventy-three percent (530/724) of neonates died in the early neonatal period, within seven days of birth. There were 147 (20.3%) deaths in the delivery room and seventy neonates (9.6%) died within the first 12 hours of admission to the neonatal ward. The various causes of neonatal death according to the PPIP classification are shown in **Figure 1**.

3.1. Birth weight

The mortality rate was strongly associated with birth weight. There were 3134 LBW neonates, with a mortality rate of 18.6% (586/3134). The majority of deaths in LBW neonates occurred in VLBW neonates (30.1% (479/1590)). Significantly more VLBW neonates died than babies >1500 g (30.1% vs. 7.1%; $p < 0.001$). The number of neonates and those who died in each birth weight category is shown in **Table 1**.

Birth weight (g)	Number	Died	% Mortality
<1000 (ELBW)	524	315	60.1
1000–1499	1066	164	15.4
1500–2499	1544	107	6.4
2500–3999 (TAGA)	1730	130	7.5
>4000 (TLGA)	154	8	5.2

Table 1. Distribution of deaths by birth weight category for neonates at CMJAH between 2013 and 2015.

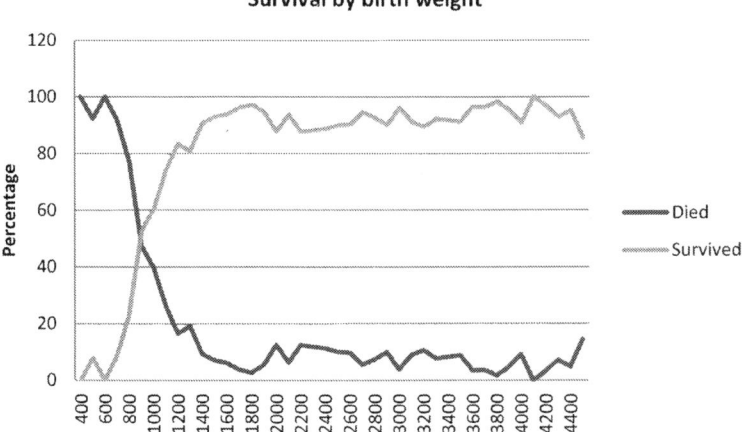

Figure 2. Percentage surviving by birth weight for neonates at CMJAH between 2013 and 2015.

The highly significant association between decreasing birth weight and increasing mortality is shown in **Figure 2** which depicts how the proportion surviving increases as birth weight increases. The percentage survival for a birth weight of 900 g is 52.8.

3.1.1. Demographic and clinical characteristics in VLBW neonates compared to bigger babies

Further results are reported for VLBW neonates compared to bigger babies. Demographic, maternal, and clinical characteristics are shown in **Table 2**. Certain conditions only occur in bigger babies and were thus not reported for VLBW neonates, namely meconium aspiration syndrome (MAS), persistent pulmonary hypertension of the neonate (PPHN), hypoxic ischemic encephalopathy (HIE), and cerebral cooling.

Factor	Cases	%	<1500 g		>1500 g		P-value
			n	%	n	%	
Birth defect	264	5.4	29	1.9	226	6.8	<0.001
Delivery room death	147	2.9	54	3.5	33	1	<0.001
Birth place							<0.001
-Other unit	718	14.4	162	10.5	552	14.5	
-Born outside health facility	194	3.9	85	5.5	104	3.8	<0.001
-Inborn	4059	81.6	1302	84.1	2707	80.5	
Antenatal care	4017	85.6	1150	77.4	2829	89	<0.001
Antenatal steroids	889	27.8	657	74.5	225	25.5	<0.001
Antenatal magnesium sulfate	102	2.3	65	4.7	37	1.2	<0.001
Chorioamnionitis	127	2.8	47	3.4	79	2.5	0.118
Maternal hypertension	651	14.3	377	27	269	8.7	<0.001
Maternal HIV	1410	29.4	456	31	946	28.9	0.147
Maternal syphilis	79	1.6	29	2.1	48	1.5	0.164
Maternal diabetes	134	2.9	7	0.5	127	4	<0.001
Maternal TB	44	1	11	0.8	33	1.1	0.416
Teenage mother	114	2.3	39	2.7	75	2.4	0.529
Vaginal delivery	2191	44.7	661	43.3	1489	44.9	0.288
Male gender	2752	55	720	46.5	1995	58.7	<0.001
Multiple gestation	586	11.8	272	17.8	301	8.9	<0.001
Delivery room resuscitation	1532	31	643	43.7	850	25	<0.001
Early onset sepsis	173	3.4	62	4.2	111	3.3	0.133
Oxygen on day 28	404	8.1	347	25.6	57	1.7	<0.001

Factor	Cases	%	<1500 g		>1500 g		P-value
			n	%	n	%	
IVH 3/4	61	1.2			N/A	N/A	
PVL	11	0.2	8	0.7	3	0.1	<0.001
Died within 12 h of admission	70	1.4	39	2.6	31	0.9	<0.001
Pneumothorax	36	0.7	10	0.7	26	0.8	0.444
Pulmonary hemorrhage	32	0.7	27	1.8	5	0.1	<0.001
HIE 2/3	174	3.6	N/A	N/A			
Cerebral cooling	103	38.1	N/A	N/A			
Meconium aspiration syndrome	264	7.8	N/A	N/A			
PPHN	54	1.6	N/A	N/A			
HMD	2004	41.1	1347	89.6	657	19.5	<0.001
NCPAP	1565	32.5	1015	70.1	550	32.5	<0.001
IPPV	692	14.4	299	21	393	11.7	<0.001
NCPAP without IPPV	1228	24.5	795	78.9	433	79.4	0.816
Surfactant therapy	1580	33.1	1038	69.8	542	16.5	<0.001
Steroids for CLD	216	5.7	199	13.8	17	0.7	<0.001
PDA	245	5	152	10.2	93	2.8	<0.001
NEC	156	3.2	107	7.2	49	1.5	<0.001
Other surgery	136	2.9	29	2	107	3.3	0.014
Packed cell transfusion	674	13.4	527	35.9	147	4.4	<0.001
Exchange transfusion	24	1.5	9	1	15	2.2	0.039
Hypoglycemia	525	10.8	185	12.3	340	10	0.02
Hyperglycemia	375	7.7	287	19.1	88	2.6	<0.001
Hypernatraemia	169	3.5	148	9.8	21	0.6	<0.001
Metabolic acidosis	185	3.8	92	6.1	93	2.8	<0.001
Late onset sepsis	608	12.6	421	28.3	187	5.6	<0.001

Table 2. Demographic, maternal and clinical characteristics by birth weight for neonates at CMJAH between 2013 and 2015.

3.2. Risk factors for neonatal death

Neonates who survived were born at a significantly more mature gestational age than those who died (34.8 weeks [SD 4.4] vs. 30.5 weeks [SD 5.5]; $p < 0.001$). Similarly, the birth weight of neonates who survived was significantly greater than those who died (2260 g [SD 932] vs. 1495 g [SD 940]; $p < 0.001$). Survivors stayed in hospital for a longer period of time than those neonates who died (14.8 days [SD 18.5] vs. 7.1 days [SD 13.3]; $p < 0.001$). Body temperature on admission was significantly higher in neonates who survived compared to those who died (36.3°C [SD8.0] vs. 35.6°C [SD 1.6]).

Conditions significantly associated with death in all the neonates, including those who died in the delivery room, are shown in **Table 3**. Only data for babies who died are reported. The percentages refer to the number of babies who died with and without the various conditions. For example, 38.5% (102) of babies who had a major birth defect died and 12.8% (596) of babies without a major birth defect died. Percentages are reported per the total number of complete cases for each condition—missing data were excluded. All other conditions were not significantly associated with death in the whole group of neonates.

Factor	Condition present		Condition absent		P
	# Died	%	# Died	%	
Birth defect	102	38.5	596	12.8	<0.001
Antenatal care	503	12.5	162	23.0	<0.001
Maternal HIV	209	14.8	433	12.8	0.061
Maternal diabetes	9	6.7	607	13.5	0.023
Vaginal delivery	404	18.4	303	11.2	<0.001
Birth place					
Another unit	100	13.9			
Outside health facility	53	27.3			<0.001
Inborn	569	34.0			
Multiple gestation	101	17.2	612	14.0	0.035
Initial resuscitation	393	25.7	312	9.2	<0.001
MAS	34	`12.9	156	5.0	<0.001
Pneumothorax	12	33.3	559	11.6	<0.001
Pulmonary haemorrhage	24	75.0	558	11.6	<0.001
PPHN	25	46.3	165	5.0	<0.001
Hyaline membrane disease	399	19.9	183	6.4	<0.001
NCPAP	304	19.4	266	8.2	<0.001
IPPV	219	31.6	348	8.5	<0.001
NCPAP without IPPV	205	16.7	98	30.2	<0.001
Surfactant therapy	310	19.6	256	8.0	<0.001

Factor	Condition present		Condition absent		P
	# Died	%	# Died	%	
PVL	4	36.4	424	9.5	0.003
IVH grade 3/4	29	47.5	32	52.5	<0.001
HIE grade 2/3	48	27.9	124	72.1	<0.001
NEC	65	41.7	508	10.9	<0.001
Surgery (not NEC)	38	27.7	524	11.4	<0.001
Blood transfusion	148	22.0	422	10.1	<0.001
Hypoglycemia	78	14.9	504	11.6	0.029
Hyperglycemia	165	44.0	417	9.3	<0.001
Hypernatraemia	64	37.9	518	11.0	<0.001
Metabolic acidosis	101	54.6	481	10.3	<0.001
Late onset sepsis	135	22.0	434	10.3	<0.001

Table 3. Factors associated with death in all neonates who died (n = 724), including delivery room deaths.

The results of binary logistic regression, considering whether neonate survived to discharge as the outcome variable, are shown in **Table 4**. The chances of survival decreased with metabolic acidosis, hyperglycemia, mechanical ventilation, major birth defect and the need for resuscitation at birth, while increasing birth weight and gestational age and delivery by Caesarean section were associated with an increased chance of survival.

Condition	Odds ratio	95% CI for OR	
		Lower	Upper
Metabolic acidosis	0.135	0.09	0.204
Hyperglycemia	0.307	0.23	0.409
Mechanical ventilation	0.357	0.278	0.46
Birth weight	1.001	1	1.001
Major birth defect	0.118	0.079	0.175
Gestational age	1.109	1.054	1.167
Caesarean section	1.803	1.444	2.251
Resuscitated at birth	0.395	0.315	0.495
Constant	0.21		

Table 4. Results of binary logistic regression model for factors associated with survival in all neonates at CMJAH between 2013 and 2015.

3.2.1. Binary logistic regression: VLBW neonates

The results of binary logistic regression considering survival to discharge as the outcome variable were performed for VLBW neonates (see **Table 5**). The percentage survival increased with increasing birth weight, delivery by Caesarean section and the use of NCPAP without the need for mechanical ventilation. Maternal HIV, hyperglycemia, resuscitation at birth, pulmonary hemorrhage, NEC, and metabolic acidosis were associated with a reduced chance of survival.

Factor	Odds ratio	95% CI	
		Lower	Upper
Birth weight (g)	1.005	1.004	1.006
Maternal HIV	0.582	0.394	0.861
Caesarean section	1.81	1.242	2.638
Resuscitated at birth	0.589	0.405	0.858
Pulmonary haemorrhage	0.176	0.063	0.493
Necrotising enterocolitis	0.252	0.139	0.459
Hyperglycaemia	0.489	0.325	0.737
Metabolic acidosis	0.098	0.051	0.191
NCPAP without ventilation	2.032	1.314	3.142
Constant	0.022		

Table 5. Binary logistic regression for factors associated with survival to discharge in VLBW neonates at CMJAH between 2013 and 2015.

3.2.2. Binary logistic regression: bigger neonates

The results of binary logistic regression considering survival to discharge as the outcome are shown in **Table 6**. Birth weight was not significantly different between survivors and non-survivors in this weight category. Decreasing gestational age, the need for resuscitation at birth, mechanical ventilation, metabolic acidosis, and hyperglycemia were all associated with a reduced chance of survival.

Factor	Odds ratio	95% CI for OR	
		Lower	Upper
Gestational age (weeks)	0.937	0.881	0.996
Resuscitated at birth	0.375	0.249	0.564
Mechanical ventilation	0.12	0.078	0.184
Metabolic acidosis	0.244	0.122	0.486
Hyperglycaemia	0.16	0.08	0.321
Constant	668.746		

Table 6. Binary logistic regression for factors associated with survival to discharge in bigger neonates at CMJAH between 2013 and 2015.

3.2.3. Delivery room deaths

Neonates who died in the delivery room were less likely to have received antenatal steroids and be delivered to mothers with hypertension or HIV, compared to neonates who died in the neonatal wards. Delivery room deaths were associated with vaginal delivery and were more likely in neonates who had been resuscitated at birth (see **Table 7**). Neonates who died in the delivery room had a lower body temperature on admission than those who died in the neonatal wards (34.6°C [SD 2.8] compared to 35.8°C [SD 1.2]; $p < 0.001$). All other variables including birth weight and gestational age were not different between neonates who died in the delivery room compared to the neonatal wards.

Condition present	Delivery room death	Percentage	Neonatal ward death	Percentage	P-value
Antenatal steroids	15	9.4	144	32.3	0.001
Maternal hypertension	12	12.2	86	17.3	0.032
Maternal HIV	25	21.6	184	35.2	0.004
Caesarean section	51	35.4	252	44.8	0.042
Resuscitated at birth	95	64.6	297	53.2	0.013

Table 7. Maternal and delivery room factors compared between babies who died in the delivery room and those who died in the neonatal wards.

4. Discussion

The ongoing audit of neonatal mortality and neonatal care to determine risk factors for poor outcome is essential so that correct interventions can be implemented. The MDG 2015 report states that better readily available data is urgently needed to guide health policies [1]. There is a slogan in the report that says "together we can measure what we treasure". The so-called "Plan Do Study Act [PDS] cycle is a tool for quality improvement projects [10]. Ongoing clinical audit is fundamental to quality improvement projects, both for planning the intervention and then measuring the benefit of the intervention [11, 12]. It is also essential to have appropriate local data available; different NICUs and neonatal populations have different problems and need tailored solutions. For example, maternal HIV is an important issue in the current study, but would not apply in a European setting.

The best example of clinical audit and quality improvement in neonatal care is the Vermont Oxford Network [VON] (www.vtoxford.org). The VON is a multinational multicenter collaboration of neonatal units established in 1989 with the aim of improving quality and effectiveness of neonatal care by research, education and quality improvement projects [13]. There are currently more than 1000 neonatal units from around the world that participate in the VON. Collaborative multi-disciplinary quality improvement projects [NIC/Q] are conducted annually [14].

The present study was an audit of neonatal survival and risk factors for poor outcome in Johannesburg, South Africa. The overall neonatal survival rate in the present study was 85.6%.

Birth weight greatly influenced survival with 69.1% of VLBW surviving compared to 92.1% of neonates above 1500 g birth weight. The VLBW survival in our unit was significantly less than that reported in the VON [www.vtoxford.org] for the same period (69.1% vs. 85.6%). Neonatal mortality rates among different neonatal units are highly variable, but the rates reported in the present study are within the reported range for developing nations [3]. The current neonatal survival rates are better than those reported from NICUs in The Gambia [4] and Ethiopia [15], but worse than those reported from a NICU in Thailand [16]. It must be noted that different mortality rates will be reported depending on which neonates are included in the audit—the present study included neonates from 400 g birth weight and those who died within the delivery room—omission of these would improve the results.

The most important causes of neonatal death in the present study were complications of prematurity, perinatal asphyxia, infection, and birth defects. These findings are similar to other studies evaluating risk factors for neonatal mortality [1, 17], although the contribution of prematurity to neonatal death is considerably higher than that reported in United Nations Millennium Development Goal Report 2015 [1] (42.3% vs. 35%). Birth weight is closely linked to gestational age in LBW neonates; the higher mortality with decreasing birth weight in the present study corresponds to increasingly premature neonates. It is interesting to note that in bigger babies, gestational age, rather than birth weight, was associated with survival. Almost 15% of deaths in the present study were due to congenital abnormalities; this reflects the fact that the unit was a referral centre for pediatric surgery; so many neonates with major congenital abnormalities were referred in for surgery.

The present results are also similar to a report from a private healthcare group in South Africa, who found that birth weight, Apgar score, and mode of delivery were all associated with neonatal mortality [18]. This is interesting, as the majority of patients in the private health care group were of White and Indian ethnicity, whereas those in the current report were almost exclusively Black African.

Most of the neonatal deaths in the current study occurred in VLBW neonates; therefore resources need to be focused on this group of neonates in order to reduce childhood mortality. Decreasing birth weight, maternal HIV, the need for resuscitation at birth, pulmonary hemorrhage, NEC, hyperglycemia, and metabolic acidosis were all associated with a decreased chance of survival in VLBW neonates, while delivery by Caesarean section and the use of NCPAP without the need for mechanical ventilation significantly increased survival. These findings are similar to reports from the same unit [5, 6]. Interventions need to be devised to address these specific risk factors, such as ensuring prevention of mother to child transmission of HIV, providing proper prompt neonatal resuscitation, maintaining normoglycemia, and promoting breastfeeding. All preterm neonates, irrespective of birth weight, should be provided with NCPAP. The use of surfactant and mechanical ventilation may not be available in all NICUs in LMICS due to resource limitations. If necessary, surfactant and mechanical ventilation can be rationed using prognostic criteria. The association of better survival with Caesarean section is a more difficult one – it is possible that neonates delivered by Caesarean section are the "better babies." These mothers may have attended antenatal care, been admitted earlier in labor, and received antenatal steroids. It is therefore possible that Caesarean section is a confounding variable. It is certainly not feasible to suggest that all preterm neonates in LMICS be delivered by Caesarean section. Other factors such as antenatal care, antenatal steroid use, and neonatal infection were not significantly predictive of survival in the present study. This does not mean, however, that regular antenatal care attendance, the use of antenatal steroids, and infection control should be omitted from interventions to improve VLBW survival.

The factors associated with poor survival in bigger neonates included decreasing gestational age, the need for resuscitation at birth, mechanical ventilation, metabolic acidosis, and hyperglycemia. This emphasizes the need for all birth attendants to be skilled in neonatal resuscitation. It is possible that mechanical ventilation will not be available in many NICUs in LIMICs, but bigger preterm infants can be successfully managed with surfactant therapy and NCPAP [9].

A recent report from Burundi showed that the neonatal survival rates were significantly improved in a low resourced district hospital, without specialist care [19]. This was achieved by integrating neonatal and obstetric services, with an emphasis on prompt referral and transfer of mothers in preterm labor, the ongoing on-site training of staff with clear protocols for case management, provision of essential equipment, and providing complementary kangaroo mother care and NICU facilities.

In conclusion, ongoing clinical audit is integral to the process of quality improvement, to develop appropriate health care policies and to monitor the impact of these policies. Focus on neonatal care and especially that of VLBW neonates is essential if we are to achieve the SDG goal of reducing neonatal mortality to 12 per 1000 births.

Author details

Daynia Elizabeth Ballot[1*] and Tobias Chirwa[2]

*Address all correspondence to: daynia.ballot@wits.ac.za

1 Department of Paediatrics and Child Health, University of the Witwatersrand, Johannesburg, South Africa

2 Division of Epidemiology and Biostatistics, School of Public Health, University of the Witwatersrand, Johannesburg, South Africa

References

[1]   United Nations. The Millenium Development Goals Report 2015. United Nations, 2015 July 2015. Report No.

[2] Kumar S, Kumar N, Vivekadhish S. Millennium Development Goals [MDGs] to Sustainable Development Goals [SDGs]: addressing unfinished agenda and strengthening sustainable development and partnership. Indian J Community Med. 2016;41[1]: 1–4.

[3] Chow S, Chow R, Popovic M, Lam M, Popovic M, Merrick J, et al. A selected review of the mortality rates of neonatal intensive care units. Front Public Health. 2015;3:225.

[4] Okomo UA, Dibbasey T, Kassama K, Lawn JE, Zaman SM, Kampmann B, et al. Neonatal admissions, quality of care and outcome: 4 years of inpatient audit data from The Gambia's teaching hospital. Paediatr Int Child Health. 2015;35[3]:252–264.

[5] Ballot DE, Chirwa TF, Cooper PA. Determinants of survival in very low birth weight neonates in a public sector hospital in Johannesburg. BMC Pediatr. 2010;10:30.

[6] Ballot DE, Chirwa T, Ramdin T, Chirwa L, Mare I, Davies VA, et al. Comparison of morbidity and mortality of very low birth weight infants in a Central Hospital in Johannesburg between 2006/2007 and 2013. BMC Pediatr. 2015;15:20.

[7] Kalimba EM BD. Survival of extremely low-birth-weight infants. S Afr J Child Health. 2013;7[1]:13–16.

[8] Harris PA, Taylor R, Thielke R, Payne J, Gonzalez N, Conde JG. Research electronic data capture [REDCap]—a metadata-driven methodology and workflow process for providing translational research informatics support. J Biomed Inform. 2009;42[2]:377–381.

[9] Jardine C, Ballot DE. The use of nasal CPAP at Charlotte Maxeke Johannesburg Academic Hospital. S Afr J Child Health. 2015;9[1]:4.

[10] Speroff T, James BC, Nelson EC, Headrick LA, Brommels M. Guidelines for appraisal and publication of PDSA quality improvement. Qual Manag Health Care. 2004;13[1]: 33–39.

[11] Dalal PG, Porath J, Parekh U, Dhar P, Wang M, Hulse M, et al. A quality improvement project to reduce hypothermia in infants undergoing MRI scanning. Pediatr Radiol. 2016.

[12] Read B, Lee DS, Fraser D. Evaluation of a practice guideline for the management of respiratory distress syndrome in preterm infants: a quality improvement initiative. Paediatr Child Health. 2016;21[1]:e4-9.

[13] Horbar JD. The Vermont Oxford Network: evidence-based quality improvement for neonatology. Pediatrics. 1999;103[1 Suppl E]:350–359.

[14] Horbar JD, Carpenter JH, Buzas J, Soll RF, Suresh G, Bracken MB, et al. Collaborative quality improvement to promote evidence based surfactant for preterm infants: a cluster randomised trial. BMJ. 2004;329[7473]:1004.

[15] Kokeb M, Desta T. Institution Based prospective cross-sectional study on patterns of neonatal morbidity at Gondar University Hospital Neonatal Unit, North-West Ethiopia. Ethiop J Health Sci. 2016;26[1]:73–79.

[16] Sritipsukho S, Suarod T, Sritipsukho P. Survival and outcome of very low birth weight infants born in a university hospital with level II NICU. J Med Assoc Thai. 2007;90[7]: 1323–1329.

[17] Dhaded SM, Somannavar MS, Vernekar SS, Goudar SS, Mwenche M, Derman R, et al. Neonatal mortality and coverage of essential newborn interventions 2010–2013: a prospective, population-based study from low-middle income countries. Reprod Health. 2015;12 Suppl 2:S6.

[18] Pepler PT, Uys DW, Nel DG. Predicting mortality and length-of-stay for neonatal admissions to private hospital neonatal intensive care units: a Southern African retrospective study. Afr Health Sci. 2012;12[2]:166–173.

[19] Ndelema B, Van den Bergh R, Manzi M, van den Boogaard W, Kosgei RJ, Zuniga I, et al. Low-tech, high impact: care for premature neonates in a district hospital in Burundi. A way forward to decrease neonatal mortality. BMC Res Notes. 2016;9[1]:28.

Chapter 7

Epidemiology of Vitamin B$_{12}$ Deficiency

Tekin Guney, Aysun Senturk Yikilmaz and
Imdat Dilek

Additional information is available at the end of the chapter

http://dx.doi.org/10.5772/63760

Abstract

Vitamin B$_{12}$ is only synthesized by microorganisms in nature and thus, is obtained by human beings through their diet. Since the most important source of vitamin B$_{12}$ is animal proteins, vegetarians may lack sufficient quantities of this vitamin in their diets. Vitamin B$_{12}$ deficiency may stem from a lower dietary intake, an autoimmune issue related to intrinsic factors or gastrointestinal system diseases resulting in vitamin B$_{12}$ malabsorption. The most important symptoms and findings of severe vitamin B$_{12}$ deficiency are anemia and neurological problems. If it is not treated, anemia symptoms and neurological disturbances resulting in spinal cord and cerebral cortex demyelination may emerge. Vitamin B$_{12}$ deficiency is one of the most frequent vitamin deficiencies worldwide. This deficiency is a highly important public health issue because of its serious complications if it is not detected and treated appropriately, although its treatment is very simple. Epidemiological studies in this field are, therefore, of great value. Most of the studies on this subject have been examined vitamin status of the general population. The research generally contains to the national or provincial populations data. Nevertheless, the few data are not fully representative in the general population. Determining risk factors and at-risk groups, and educating them about vitamin B$_{12}$ deficiency and proper diet would prevent the irreversible complications of this type of deficiency. The goal of this study is to review epidemiological studies related to vitamin B$_{12}$ deficiency and to point out the importance of identifying and treating it.

Keywords: epidemiology, vitamin B$_{12}$, anemia, deficiency, nutrition

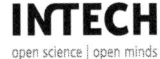

1. Introduction

Vitamin B_{12} is only synthesized by microorganisms in nature and thus, is obtained by human beings through their diet [1]. Since the most important source of vitamin B_{12} is animal proteins, vegetarians may lack sufficient quantities of this vitamin in their diets.

Vitamin B_{12} deficiency may be caused by a lower dietary intake (impaired absorption or decreased intake), an autoimmune issue related to intrinsic factors or gastrointestinal system diseases resulting in vitamin B_{12} malabsorption [2]. The most important symptoms and findings of severe vitamin B_{12} deficiency are anemia and neurological problems. Vitamin B_{12} deficiency is one of the most common causes of macrocytic anemia [3, 4]. If it is not treated, anemia symptoms and neurological disturbances resulting in spinal cord and cerebral cortex demyelination may emerge [5].

Epidemiology concerns health and disorders, etiological agents, the symptoms of disorders, diagnoses and the benefits of clinical care, and its discontinuation. Determining risk factors and at-risk groups as well as educating them about vitamin B_{12} deficiency, proper diet, and replacement would prevent any irreversible complications of this type of deficiency. The goal of this study is to review epidemiological studies related to vitamin B_{12} deficiency and to point out the importance of identifying and treating it.

2. The metabolism of vitamin B_{12}

The major metabolic pathway of vitamin B_{12} formation is shown in **Figure 1**.

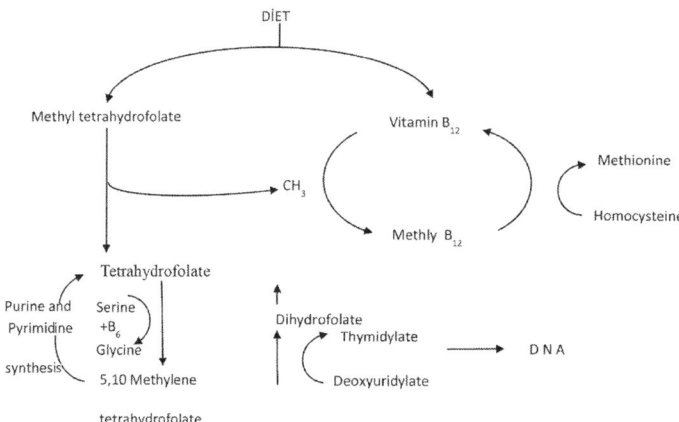

Figure 1. The mechanism of vitamin B_{12}.

Vitamin B_{12} is essential for DNA synthesis in cells. It has two different forms in cells.

Deoxyadenosyl B$_{12}$ converts methylmalonyl CoA to succinyl CoA. It also transfers methyl groups from methyltetrafolate to synthesized methionine. Transferring a methyl group from methyltetrafolate forms tetrahydrofolate. If there is a lack of vitamin B$_{12}$, there is no receptor to transfer a methyl group from methyltetrafolate. Then the methylfolate is trapped and tetrahydrofolate that is needed to support DNA synthesis is decreased [2].

3. The absorption and distribution of vitamin B$_{12}$

The absorption of vitamin B$_{12}$ is a multiple staged process. Vitamin B$_{12}$ intake through dietary sources initially combines with binding proteins (R-protein) in the saliva. Then it reaches the intestine where pancreatic protease is extracted and it combines with intrinsic factors which contain glycoprotein. Vitamin B$_{12}$ is absorbed efficiently when it combines with such intrinsic factors. In fact, very little uncombined free vitamin B$_{12}$ is absorbed. The vitamin B$_{12}$ and intrinsic factor binds with a specific receptor on the mucosa cells of the terminal ileum and is extracted to the circulation system from the intestine wall. Vitamin B$_{12}$ is bound with transcobalamin proteins in circulation. The most important transcobalamin protein is transcobalamin II that is the main transporter protein in distributing vitamin B$_{12}$ to the tissues and liver [5].

Tissues rich in vitamin B$_{12}$ include parenchymal tissues (above 100 mcg/100 g), fish, muscular organs, dairy products, and egg yolks (1–10 mcg/100 g) [5]. In the West, daily vitamin B$_{12}$ intake by nonvegetarians is approximately 5–7 mcg/day, which is sufficient for normal homeostasis of body functions [6]. However, vegetarians are at risk of vitamin B$_{12}$ deficiency because they only consume 0.25–0.5 mcg/day vitamin B$_{12}$ from their diet [6]. Vitamin B$_{12}$ is stored well in tissues; for adults, vitamin B$_{12}$ levels are 2–5 mg and this is mostly located in the liver (approximately 1 mg). Daily loss of vitamin B$_{12}$ level is 0.1%. When someone no longer obtains vitamin B$_{12}$ through their diet, depletion of the stored vitamin may take as long as 3–4 years [6].

4. The clinical spectrum of vitamin B$_{12}$ deficiency

Both vitamin B$_{12}$ deficiency and folate deficiency cause megaloblastic anemia. In fact, only vitamin B$_{12}$ deficiency causes neuorological change. Additionally, the difference between these two anemia types is the duration between the start of deficiency and symptoms being apparent. The symptoms of B$_{12}$ deficiency appear within years after the removal of vitamin B$_{12}$ from the diet whereas the symptoms of folate deficiency are seen within 4–6 weeks.

Vitamin B$_{12}$ deficiency is one of the most frequent vitamin deficiencies worldwide [7]. So, this deficiency is an extremely important public health issue owing to its serious complications if it is not detected and treated appropriately. Epidemiological studies in this field are, therefore, of great value. There are many epidemiological studies related to vitamin B$_{12}$ deficiency, which have used different methods and evaluated different disorders accompanying it [8, 9].

5. The epidemiology of vitamin B$_{12}$ deficiency

Although vitamin B$_{12}$ deficiency is considered to be a public health problem, its incidence and prevalence are not exactly known. The reasons for this condition are the ethnic and sociocultural differences between societies and their varying dietary habits. The most comprehensive knowledge about vitamin B$_{12}$ deficiency has been extracted from a review, which was conducted through studies in Africa, America, South-East Asia, Europe, Eastern Mediterranean, and Western Pacific in 2008 [10]. Another review evaluated 41 studies in Latin America and the Caribbean and found that the prevalence of vitamin B$_{12}$ deficiency was 61% [11].

The data extracted from this study have shown that vitamin B$_{12}$ deficiency is still a public health problem in these regions. The main reasons for vitamin B$_{12}$ deficiency are nutritional deficiencies that affect large sectors of the population including vegetarians and their children who are affected during and after pregnancy, the elderly, frequent drug users as well as nutritional deficiency linked to low socioeconomic level [12].

Vitamin B$_{12}$ deficiency among vegetarians was found to be between 21 and 85% regardless of age, address, type of vegetarianism, and demographics of the individuals concerned (**Table 1**) [13].

Although it is thought that vitamin B$_{12}$ deficiency is rarely seen except in strict vegetarians, it is, in fact, commonly seen in all vegetarian groups (lacto-vegetarians, ovo-vegetarians, lacto-ovo-vegetarians, and vegans), as well as among the elderly and for reasons related to medicine and drug use [13–16]. Particularly, vegetarians should take care of protective measures for vitamin B$_{12}$ deficiency that involve to identify the inadequate vitamin level and to receive supplements containing B$_{12}$ in necessary condition [13].

Reference	Country	Participants	Rate of deficiency
Dhonukshe-Rutten et al. [17]	Netherlands	$N = 73$, age range : 9–15 years	41%
Donaldson [18]	USA	$N = 49$, mean age : 55 years	47%
Geisel et al. [19]	Germany	$N = 71$, mean age : 53–51 years	58%
Gibson et al. [20]	Ethiopia	$N = 99$, mean age : 27.8 years	62%
Gilsing et al. [21]	UK	$N = 65$, mean age : 42.8 years	40%
Hermann et al. [22]	Germany and Netherlands	$N = 111$, mean age : 46 years	55%

Reference	Country	Participants	Rate of deficiency
Hermann et al. [23]	Oman (German and Asian-Indian immigrants)	N = 96, mean age : 50 years	66% of German and 69% of Indians
Hermann et al. [24]	Germany	N = 34, mean age : 22 years	43%
Hermann et al. [25]	Germany and Netherland	N = 66, mean age : 48 years	73%
Hermann et al. [26]	Germany	N = 114, mean age : 50 years	74%
Kwok et al. [27]	China	N = 119, mean age : >55 years	42%
Kwok et al. [28]	Hong Kong	N = 113, mean age : >55 years	81%
Miller et al. [29]	USA	N = 110, adults (21–70 years) N = 42, children	30% 55%
Obeid et al. [30]	Germany and Netherland	N = 111	Unclear. Figure shows 58% but text reports 85%
Refsum et al. [31]	India	N = 78 (27–55 years)	75%
Rush et al. [32]	New Zealand	N = 6 (9–11 years)	50%
Schneede et al. [33]	Norway	N = 41, infants (11.4–21.9 months)	85.4%
van Dusseldorp et al. [34]	Netherlands	N = 73, adolescents (9–15 years)	21%

Table 1. Studies into vitamin B$_{12}$ deficiency and vegetarianism [13].

The effects of vitamin B$_{12}$ on the central nervous system are well known. Lifelong optimal vitamin B$_{12}$ levels are very important for cognitive function. Vitamin B$_{12}$ deficiency that is caused by suboptimal vitamin B$_{12}$ intake and/or changes in absorption due to aging, directly causes neurocognitive deficiencies by neurotoxic effect [35, 36]. Several epidemiological studies about vitamin B$_{12}$ and the effects of aging on cognitive function have found a correlation between vitamin B$_{12}$ and cognitive function among middle-aged and elderly cases in Central and Eastern Europe [37].

Another study which researched vitamin B_{12} prevalence among the middle-aged and elderly in Europe reported vitamin B_{12} deficiency to be between 5 and 46% [38–40].

Vitamin B_{12} deficiency resulting from drug use has been shown in several previous studies and indeed is still being discussed. Especially, metformin, which is used to treat diabetes mellitus type-2 (DM), influences vitamin B_{12} absorption by affecting the calcium-dependent ileal absorption of intrinsic factor-vitamin B_{12} complex [41, 42].

However, there are studies which defend the contrary [42, 43]. Neither intestinal motility changes nor bacterial over reproduction could be shown in these studies. The relationship between vitamin B_{12} absorption and metformin was first observed in 30% of type-2 diabetic patients in 1971, and Ting et al. also found a relationship between vitamin B_{12} and the use of metformin in treatment doses in 2006 [16, 44].

Vitamin B_{12} deficiency related with the use of metformin was observed among 30 patients, 90% of whom had minor hematological abnormalities, 30% had mild peripheral neuropathy, and two patients had symptomatic anemia and pancytopenia [45].

A meta-analysis, which evaluated six randomized controlled trials, found that using metformin in different doses caused vitamin B_{12} deficiency and there was a correlation between the metformin dosage and level of vitamin B_{12} deficiency [46].

Levodopa is another drug which is used for parkinsonism and believed to cause vitamin B_{12} deficiency. Levodopa has an effect on vitamin B_{12} levels by affecting the catechol-O-methyl transferase pathway and carbidopa metabolism [47–49]. According to these studies, vitamin B_{12} levels should be checked before planning to use metformin and levodopa for a long-term period.

The prevalence of vitamin B_{12} deficiency was reported to be very high over the last decade that is why national programs have been established to prevent it [50, 51].

Consequently, vitamin B_{12} deficiency has been found to be very common in specific groups of the population, and there is a high risk of vitamin B_{12} deficiency as far as vegetarians, infants, pregnant and breastfeeding mothers, and the elderly are concerned. There is clearly a need to establish both national and prophylaxis programs in order to prevent vitamin B_{12} deficiency among such cases.

Author details

Tekin Guney[1*], Aysun Senturk Yikilmaz[2] and Imdat Dilek[2]

*Address all correspondence to: tekin-guney@hotmail.com

1 Department of Hematology, Turkiye Yuksek Ihtisas Training and Research Hospital, Ankara, Turkey

2 Department of Hematology, Yildirim Beyazit University Medical Faculty, Ankara, Turkey

References

[1] Carmel R: Biomarkers of cobalamin (vitamin B-12) status in the epidemiologic setting: a critical overview of context, applications, and performance characteristics of cobalamin, methylmalonicacid, and holotranscobalamin II. Am J Clin Nutr.2011;94:348S–358S.

[2] Hillman RS, Ault KA, Rinder HM (translation editors: Haznedaroglu IC, Turgut M, Buyukasik Y, Goker H). Makrositik Anemiler: Klinik Pratikte Hematoloji. 4th ed.; 2009. p. 95–109.

[3] Pruthi RK, Tefferi A. Pernicious anemia are visited. Mayo Clin Proc. 1994;69:144–50.

[4] Allen RH, Stabler SP, Savage DG, Lindenbaum J. Metabolic abnormalities in cobalamin (vitamin B12) and folate deficiency. FASEB J. 1993;7:1344–53.

[5] Antony AC. Megaloblastic anemias. In: Hoffman R, Benz E, Silberstein L, Heslop H, Weitz J, Anastasi J, editors. Hematology: Basic Principles and Practice. 6th ed. Philadelphia, PA, USA: Elsevier; 2013. p. 473–504.

[6] Green R, Kinsella LJ. Current concepts in the diagnosis of cobalamin deficiency. Neurology. 1995;45:1435–40.

[7] World Health Organization, 2004. Focusing on anaemia: towards an integrated approach for effective anaemia control. http://www.who.int/nutrition/publications/micronutrients/WHOandUNICEF_statement_anaemia_en.pdf?ua=1 (accessed 26 March 2016).

[8] Liu Q, Li S, Quan H, Li J. Vitamin B12 status in metformin treated patients: systematic review. PLoS One. 2014;9(6):e100379.

[9] Bermejo F, Algaba A, Guerra I, et al. Should we monitor vitamin B12 and folate levels in Crohn's disease patients? Scand J Gastroenterol. 2013;48(11): 1272–7.

[10] McLean E, de Benoist B, Allen LH. Review of the magnitude of folate and vitamin B12 deficiencies worldwide. Food Nutr Bull. 2008;29(2 Suppl):S38–51.

[11] Brito A, Mujica-Coopman MF, López de Romaña D, Cori H, Allen LH. Folate and vitamin B12 status in Latin America and the Caribbean: an update. Food Nutr Bull. 2015;36(2 Suppl):S109–18.

[12] Hemmer B, Glocker FX, Schumacher M, et al. Subacute combined degeneration: clinical, electrophysiological, and magnetic resonance imaging findings. J Neurol Neurosurg Psychiatry. 1998;65:822–7.

[13] Pawlak R, Parrott SJ, Raj S, Cullum-Dugan D, Lucus D. How prevalent is vitamin B12 deficiency among vegetarians? Nutr. Rev. 2013;71(2):110–7.

[14]   Allen LH. How common is vitamin B12 deficiency? Am J Clin Nutr. 2009;89(Suppl):S693–96.

[15]   Stabler SP, Allen RH. Vitamin B12 deficiency as a world-wide problem. Annu Rev Nutr. 2004;24:299–326.

[16]   Ting RZ, Szeto CC, Chan MH, Ma KK, Chow KM. Risk factors of vitamin B12 deficiency in patients receiving metformin. Arch Intern Med. 2006;166(18):1975–79.

[17]   Dhonukshe-Rutten RA, van Dusseldorp M, Schneede J, et al. Low bone mineral density and bone mineral content are associated with low cobalamin status in adolescents. Eur J Nutr. 2005;44:341–47.

[18]   Donaldson MS. Metabolic vitamin B12 status on a mostly raw vegan diet with follow-up using tablets, nutritional yeast, or probiotic supplements. Ann Nutr Metab. 2000;44:229–34.

[19]   Geisel J, Schorr H, Bodis M, et al. The vegetarian lifestyle and DNA methylation. Clin Chem Lab Med. 2005;43:1164–69.

[20]   Gibson RS, Abebe Y, Stabler S, et al. Zinc, gravida, infection, and iron, but not vitamin B-12 or folate status, predict hemoglobin during pregnancy in Southern Ethiopia. J Nutr. 2008;138;581–86.

[21]   Gilsing AM, Crowe FL, Lloyd-Wright Z, et al. Serum concentrations of vitamin B12 and folate in British male omnivores, vegetarians and vegans: results from a cross-sectional analysis of the EPIC-Oxford cohort study. Eur J Clin Nutr. 2010;64:933–39.

[22]   Hermann W, Obeid R, Schorr H, et al. Functional vitamin B12 deficiency and determination of holotranscobalamin in populations at risk. Clin Chem Lab Med. 2003;41:1478–88.

[23]   Hermann W, Obeid R, Schorr H, et al. Enhanced bone metabolism in vegetarians—the role of vitamin B12 deficiency. Clin Chem Lab Med. 2009;47:1381–87.

[24]   Hermann W, Schorr H, Purschwitz K, et al. Total homocysteine, vitamin B12, and total antioxidant status in vegetarians. Clin Chem. 2001;47:1094–1101.

[25]   Hermann W, Schorr H, Obeid R, et al. Vitamin B12 status, particularly holotranscobalamin II and methylmalonic acid concentrations, and hyperhomocysteinemia in vegetarians. Am J Clin Nutr. 2003;78:131–36.

[26]   Hermann W, Obeid R, Schorr H, et al. The usefulness of holotranscobalamin in predicting vitamin B12 status in different clinical settings. Curr Drug Metab. 2005;6:47–53.

[27]   Kwok T, Cheng G, Woo J, et al. Independent effect of vitamin B12 deficiency on hematological status in older Chinese vegetarian women. Am J Hematol. 2002;70:186–90.

[28] Kwok T, Cheng G, Lai WK, et al. Use of fasting urinary methylmalonic acid to screen for metabolic vitamin B12 deficiency in older persons. Nutrition. 2004;20:764–8.

[29] Miller DR, Specker BL, Ho ML, et al. Vitamin B-12 status in a macrobiotic community. Am J Clin Nutr. 1991;53:524–9.

[30] Obeid R, Geisel J, Schorr H, et al. The impact of vegetarianism on some haematological parameters. Eur J Haematol. 2002;69:275–9.

[31] Refsum H, Yajnik CS, Gadkari M, et al. Hyperhomocysteinemia and elevated methylmalonic acid indicate a high prevalence of cobalamin deficiency in Asian Indians. Am J Clin Nutr. 2001;74:233–41.

[32] Rush EC, Chhichhia P, Hinckson E, et al. Dietary patterns and vitamin B12 status of migrants Indian preadolescent girls. Eur J Clin Nutr. 2009;63:585–7.

[33] Schneede J, Dagnelie PC, van Staveren WA, et al. Methylmalonic acid and homocysteine in plasma as indicators of functional cobalamin deficiency in infants on macrobiotic diets. Pediatr Res. 1994;36:194–201.

[34] Van Dusseldorp M, Schneede J, Refsum H, et al. Risk of persistent cobalamin deficiency in adolescents fed a macrobiotic diet in early life. Am J Clin Nutr. 1999;69:664–71.

[35] Reynolds E. Vitamin B12, folic acid, and the nervous system. Lancet Neurol. 2006;5:949–60.

[36] Allen LH. Causes of vitamin B12 and folate deficiency. Food Nutr Bull. 2008;29:20–34.

[37] Horvat P, Gardiner J, Kubinova, Pajak A, Tamosiunas A, Schöttker B, Pikhart H, Peasey A, Jansen E, Bobak M. Serum folate, vitamin B-12 and cognitive function in middle and older age: the HAPIEE study. Exp Gerontol. 2016;76:33–38.

[38] Joosten E, van der Berg A, Riezler R, Naurath HJ, Lindenbaum J et al. Metabolic evidence that deficiencies of vitamin B-12 (cobalamin), folate, and vitamin B-6 occur commonly in elderly people. Am J Clin Nutr. 1993;58:468–76.

[39] Bates CJ, Schneede J, Mishra G, Prentice A, Mansoor MA. Relationship between methylmalonic acid, homocysteine, vitamin B12 intake and status and socio-economic indices, in a subset of participants in the British National Diet and Nutrition Survey of people aged 65 y and over. Eur J Clin Nutr. 2003;57:349–57.

[40] Clarke R, Refsum H, Birks J, Evans JG, Johnston C et al. Screening for vitamin B-12 and folate deficiency in older persons. Am J Clin Nutr. 2003;77:1241–7.

[41] Snow CF. Laboratory diagnosis of vitamin B12 and folate deficiency: a guide for the primary care physician. Arch Intern Med. 1999;159:1289–98.

[42]   Bauman WA, Shaw S, Jayatilleke ES, Spungen AM, Herbert V. Increased intake of calcium reverses vitamin B12 malabsorption induced by metformin. Diabetes Care. 2000;23:1227–31.

[43]   Scarpello JH, Hodgson E, Howlett HC. Effect of metformin on bile salt circulation and intestinal motility in type 2 diabetes mellitus. Diabet Med. 1998;15(8):651–6.

[44]   Tomkin GH, Hadden DR, Weaver JA, Montgomery DA. Vitamin-B12 status of patients on long-term metformin therapy. Br Med J. 1971;19;2(5763):685–7.

[45]   Andrès E, Federici L. Vitamin B12 deficiency in patients receiving metformin: clinical data. Arch Intern Med. 2007;167(7):729.

[46]   Liu Q, Li S, Quan H, Li J. Vitamin B12 status in metformin treated patients: systematic review. PLoS One. 2014; 24;9(6):e100379.

[47]   Rajabally YA, Martey J. Neuropathy in Parkinson disease: prevalence and determinants. Neurology. 2011;77(22):1947–50.

[48]   Ceravolo R, Cossu G, Bandettini di Poggio M, et al. Neuropathy and levodopa in Parkinson's disease: evidence from a multicenter study. Mov Disord. 2013;28(10):1391–7.

[49]   Müller T, van Laar T, Cornblath DR, Odin P, Klostermann F, Grandas FJ, Ebersbach G, Urban PP, Valldeoriola F, Antonini A. Peripheral neuropathy in Parkinson's disease: levodopa exposure and implications for duodenal delivery Parkinsonism Relat Disord. 2013;19(5):501–7.

[50]   Allen LH. Folate and vitamin B12 status in the Americas. Nutr Rev. 2004;62:29–33.

[51]   McLean E, de Benoist B, Allen LH. Review of the magnitude of folate and vitamin B12 deficiencies worldwide. Food Nutr Bull. 2008;29:38–51.

β-Thalassemia: Genotypes and Phenotypes

Tamer Hassan, Mohamed Badr, Usama El Safy,

Mervat Hesham, Laila Sherief and Marwa Zakaria

Additional information is available at the end of the chapter

http://dx.doi.org/10.5772/64644

Abstract

β-Thalassemias are extremely heterogeneous at the molecular level. More than 200 disease-causing mutations have been identified. The majority of mutations are single nucleotide substitutions. Rarely, β-thalassemia results from gross gene deletion. The degree of globin chain imbalance is determined by the nature of the mutation of the β-gene. β^0 refers to the complete absence of production of β-globin on the affected allele. β^+ refers to alleles with some residual production of β-globin (around 10%). In β^{++}, the reduction in β-globin production is very mild. The broad spectrum of β-thalassemia alleles can produce a wide spectrum of different β-thalassemia phenotypes. In this chapter, we review the molecular basis of the marked heterogeneity of the thalassemia syndromes or in other words the genotype-phenotype relationship in β-thalassemia.

Keywords: β-Thalassemia, genotype, phenotype, mutation, disease

1. Introduction

β-Thalassemia syndromes are a group of hereditary blood disorders characterized by reduced or absent β-globin chain synthesis, resulting in reduced Hb in red blood cells (RBCs), decreased RBC production, and anemia. β-Thalassemia includes three main forms: Thalassemia Major, variably referred to as "Cooley's Anemia" and "Mediterranean Anemia," Thalassemia Intermedia, and Thalassemia Minor also called "β-thalassemia carrier," " β-thalassemia trait," or "heterozygous β-thalassemia" [1].

The β-thalassemia syndromes are much more diverse than the α-thalassemia syndromes due to the diversity of the mutations that produce the defects in the β-globin gene. The severity of β-thalassemia relates to the degree of imbalance between the α- and non-α-globin chains. The

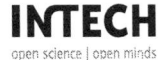

β-globin gene maps in the short arm of chromosome 11, in a region that contains also the delta globin gene, the embryonic epsilon gene, the fetal gamma genes, and a pseudogene (ψB1) [1].

Unlike the deletions that constitute most of the α-thalassemia syndromes, β-thalassemias are caused by hundreds of mutations that affect all aspects of β-globin production: transcription, translation, and the stability of the β-globin product [2].

2. Classification of β-thalassemias

1. **β-Thalassemia**

    - Thalassemia major

    - Thalassemia intermediate

    - Thalassemia minor

2. **β-Thalassemia with associated Hb anomalies**

    - HbC/β-thalassemia

    - HbE/β-thalassemia

    - HbS/β-thalassemia

3. **Hereditary persistence of fetal Hb and β-thalassemia**

4. **Autosomal dominant forms of β-thalassemia**

5. **β-Thalassemia associated with other manifestations**

    - β-Thalassemia-trichothiodystrophy

    - X-linked thrombocytopenia with thalassemia

2.1. Epidemiology of β-thalassemias

The frequency of β-thalassemia varies widely, depending on the ethnic population. The disease is reported most commonly in Mediterranean, African, and Southeast Asian populations. The highest carrier frequency is reported in Cyprus (14%), Sardinia (10.3%), and Southeast Asia [1].

Population migration and intermarriage between different ethnicities have introduced thalassemia in almost every country of the world, including Northern Europe, where thalassemia was previously absent [2].

About 1.5% of the global population (80–90 million) are β-thalassemia carriers, with about 60,000 symptomatic individuals born annually. Incidence of symptomatic individuals is estimated at 1 in 100,000 worldwide and 1 in 10,000 in Europe [2].

It is the most common chronic hemolytic anemia in Egypt (85.1%), and its carrier rate has been estimated at 9–10.2% from an examination of 1000 normal random subjects from different geographic areas of the country [3].

2.2. Etiology of β-thalassemia

β-Thalassemia is inherited as an autosomal recessive disorder. There are hundreds of mutations within the β-globin gene, but approximately 20 different alleles comprise 80% of the mutations found worldwide. Within each geographic population, there are unique mutations. The large majority of mutations are point mutations. Deletions of β-globin gene are uncommon. Mutations in β-globin gene cause a reduced or absent production of the β-globin chains [4]. **Table 1** displays the list of common mutations according to severity and ethnic distribution.

β-Gene mutation	Ethnicity	Severity
−619 del	Indian	β^0
−101 C→T	Mediterranean	β^{++}
−88 C→T	Black	β^{++}
−87 C→G	Mediterranean, African	β^{++}
−31 A→G	Japanese	β^{++}
−29 A→G	African	β^{++}
−28 A→C	Southeast Asian	β^{++}
IVS1-nt1 G→A	Mediterranean, Asian Indian	β^0
IVS1-nt5 G→C	East Asian, Asian Indian	β^0
IVS1-nt6 T→C	Mediterranean	$\beta^{+/++}$
IVS1-nt110 G→A	Mediterranean	β^+
IVS2-nt654 C→T	Chinese	β^+
IVS2-nt745 C→G	Mediterranean	β^+
Codon 39 C→T	Mediterranean	β^0
Codon 5 -CT	Mediterranean	β^0
Codon 6 -A	Mediterranean, African-American	β^0
Codon 41/42 -TTCT	Southeast Asian	β^0
AATAAA to AACAAA	African-American	β^{++}
AATAAA to AATGAA	Mediterranean	β^{++}
Codon 27 G→T Hb (Hb Knossos)	Mediterranean	β^{++}
Codon 79 G>A (Hb E)	Southeast Asian	β^{++}
Codon 19 G>A (Hb Malay)	Malaysian	

Table 1. Common mutations of β-thalassemia according to severity and ethnicity.

3. Genotype phenotype relationship in β-thalassemia

Mutations causing thalassemia can affect any step in the pathway of globin gene expression. The most common forms arise from mutations that derange splicing of the mRNA precursors or prematurely terminate translation of the mRNA. The resulting phenotype reflect the effects of the β^0 thalassemia in which there is no B-globin gene production and B^+, B^{++} thalassemia in which there is marked or mild reduction in production of β-chain [5].

3.1. Genetic modifiers

Several modifier genes have been identified which are able to influence the severity of β-thalassemia, so at phenotypic level β-thalassemias are considered multigenic diseases. Improved understanding of the influence of modifier genes involved in modulating the complex pathophysiology of β-thalassemia may allow prediction of disease phenotype [6].

3.1.1. Primary modifiers

Primary genetic modifiers in homozygous β-thalassemia include genetic variants able to reduce the globin chain imbalance, therefore resulting in a milder form of thalassemia.

1. The presence of silent or mild β-thalassemia alleles associated with a high residual output of β-globin.

2. The coinheritance of α-thalassemia.

3. Genetic determinants able to sustain a continuous production of gamma globin chains (HbF) in adult life.

3.1.2. Secondary modifiers

The clinical phenotype of homozygous β-thalassemia may also be modified by the coinheritance of other genetic variants mapping outside the globin clusters.

1. TA_7 polymorphism in the promoter region of the uridine diphosphate-glucuronosyl transferase gene is associated with cholelitiasis in thalassemic patients [7].

2. Apolipoprotein Eε4 allele seems to be a genetic risk factor for left ventricular failure in β-thalassemia [8].

3. Genes involved in iron (i.e., C282Y and H63D HFE gene mutations) and bone metabolism [9].

4. Glutathione-S-transferase M1 gene polymorphism has been associated with an increased risk of cardiac iron overload in patients with thalassemia major [10].

5. Excess functional α-globin genes (α gene triplication or quadruplicating) in heterozygous β-thalassemia may lead to thalassemia intermedia phenotype instead of the asymptomatic carrier state [11].

4. Pathophysiology of β-thalassemia

The basic defect in β-thalassemia is a reduced or absent production of β-globin chains with relative excess of α-chains. Because α- and non-α chains pair with each other at a ratio close to 1:1 to form normal Hb, the excess unmatched α chains accumulate in the cell as an unstable product, leading to cell destruction in the bone marrow and in the extramedullary sites. This process is referred to as ineffective erythropoiesis (IE) and is the hallmark of β-thalassemia [12].

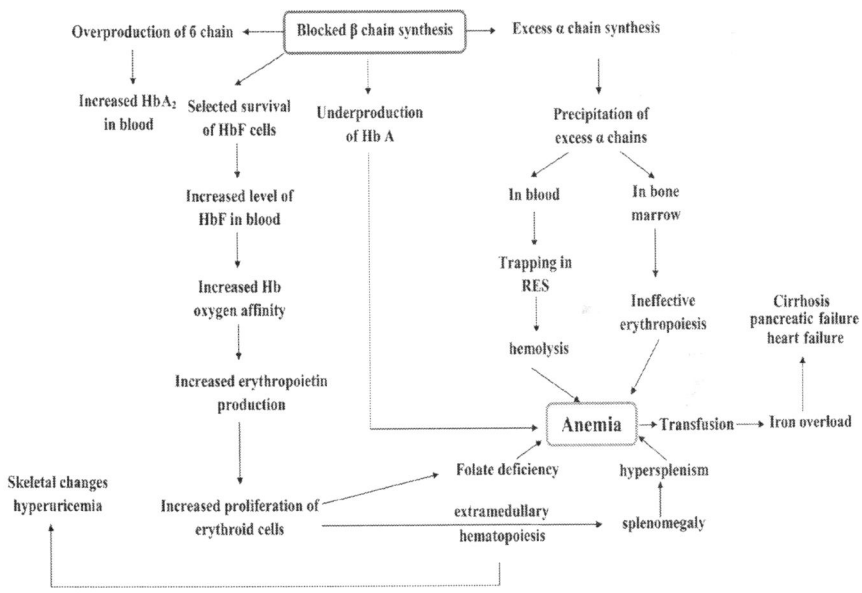

Figure 1. Pathophysiology of β-thalassemia.

The excess α-chains may, in minor amounts, combine with residual β- (in β+ -thalassemia) and γ-chains (whose synthesis persists usually in small quantity after birth), undergo proteolysis, or in large part become associated with the erythroid precursors with deleterious effects on erythroid maturation and survival. Also excess α-chain precipitation in the red cell membrane causes structural and functional alterations with changes in deformability, stability, and red cell hydration [12].

Alterations of erythroid precursors result in an enhanced rate of apoptosis, which is a programmed cell death. Apoptosis could contribute significantly to ineffective erythropoiesis and occurs primarily at the polychromatophilic erythroblast stage. The ineffective erythropoiesis (IE) and anemia have several consequences producing the clinical picture of the disease. The first response to anemia is an increased production of erythropoietin, causing a marked erythroid hyperplasia, which may range between 25 and 30 times normal. Anemia may produce cardiac enlargement and sometimes severe cardiac failure [12].

Increased erythropoietin synthesis may stimulate the formation of extramedullary erythropoietic tissue, primarily in the thorax and paraspinal region. Marrow expansion also results in characteristic deformities of the skull and face, as well as osteopenia [13].

High levels of iron, closely associated with denatured hemoglobin, have been found in the membrane of β-thalassemic red cells [14].

Severe IE, chronic anemia, and hypoxia also cause increased gastrointestinal (GI) tract iron absorption. This is combined with increased iron from the breakdown of RBCs and the increased iron introduced into the circulation by the transfusions necessary to treat thalassemia, plus inadequate excretory pathways lead to progressive deposition of iron in tissues and hemosiderosis occurs [13].

Free iron species, such as labile plasma iron as well as labile iron pool in the RBCs accumulate when transferrin saturation exceeds 70%. These free iron species generate reactive oxygen species with eventual tissue damage, organ dysfunction, and death (**Figure 1**) [13].

5. Clinical presentation of β-thalassemia

5.1. History

The history in patients with thalassemia widely varies, depending on the severity of the condition and the age at the time of diagnosis. In most patients with thalassemia traits, no unusual signs or symptoms are encountered, children with thalassemia major usually present between 3 months and 1 year of life, and occasionally presentation is delayed to 4–5 years [15].

Some patients, especially those with somewhat more severe forms of the disease, manifest some pallor and slight icteric discoloration of the sclerae with splenomegaly, leading to slight enlargement of the abdomen. Thalassemia should be considered in any child with hypochromic microcytic anemia that does not respond to iron supplementation [15].

5.2. Physical

Patients with thalassemia minor are often asymptomatic. They have mild anemia and their Hb level is usually not less than 9–10 g/dl therefore pallor and splenomegaly are rarely observed.

The stigmata of severe untreated α-thalassemia major included the following:

- Severe anemia, with an Hb level of 3–7 g/dl
- Massive hepatosplenomegaly
- Severe growth retardation
- Bony deformities

Patients with signs of iron overload may also demonstrate signs of cardiomyopathy and endocrinopathy caused by iron deposits. Diabetes and thyroid or adrenal disorders have been described in these patients [16].

6. β-Thalassemia workup

6.1. Laboratory studies

6.1.1. Complete blood count and peripheral blood film examination

In the severe forms of thalassemia, the Hb level ranges from 2 to 8 g/dl. MCV and MCH are significantly low. Reticulocyte count is elevated to 5–8% and leukocytosis is usually present. Platelet count is usually normal, unless the spleen is markedly enlarged. Peripheral blood film examination reveals nucleated RBCs and occasional immature leukocytes.

6.1.2. Hemoglobin electrophoresis

High performance liquid chromatography (HPLC) is now usually used as first-line method to diagnose hemoglobin disorders. HPLC or hemoglobin electrophoresis reveals absence or almost complete absence of Hb A, with almost all the circulating hemoglobin being Hb F. The Hb A2 percentage is normal, low, or slightly raised.

6.1.3. Biochemical studies

1. **Serum iron and ferritin:** Serum iron level and ferritin levels are elevated. However, an assessment using serum ferritin levels may underestimate the iron concentration in the liver. Liver iron concentration (LIC) could be estimated by liver biopsy or T2* MRI, which provides a noninvasive alternative to liver biopsy. LIC could also monitored by the use of superconducting quantum interference device (SQUID).

2. **Transferrin saturation:** Transferrin saturation is a surrogate marker for NTBI [17]. Transferrin saturation >50% is suggestive of a high iron load.

3. **NTBI and LPI:** NTBI and LPI are very specific for iron overload and can be used to monitor the response to chelation therapy [18].

4. **Hepcidin measurement:** Hepcidin can be measured in serum and urine using mass spectrometry, and this may be a feasible marker in the near future [19].

5. **Other biochemical changes:** Serum zinc, serum and leucocytic ascorbic acid, vitamin E, and folic acid are low. LDL is elevated as consequence of ineffective erythropoiesis [20].

6.2. Imaging studies

Findings show skeletal changes, including thinning of the cortex, widening of the medulla, and coarsening of trabeculations, due to bone marrow hyperplasia in the long bones, metacarpals, and metatarsals. Skull bones show "hair-on-end." The maxilla may overgrow, which results in maxillary overbite, prominence of the upper incisors, and separation of the orbit. These changes contribute to the classic chipmunk facies observed in patients with thalassemia major [21]. Chest radiography is used to evaluate cardiac size and shape. Left ventricular function can be quantified using MRI, MUGA (multiple gated acquisition scan) or echocardiography [22].

Cardiac T2*, a noninvasive procedure involves measuring the cardiac T2 with cardiac magnetic resonance (CMR). This procedure has shown decreased values in cardiac T2 due to iron deposit in the heart. Unlike liver MRI, CMR does not correlate well with the ferritin level, the liver iron level, or echocardiography findings. The liver is clear of iron loading much earlier than the heart, and so the decision to stop or reduce chelation treatment based on liver iron levels is misleading [23].

A poor correlation was noted between cardiac and hepatic iron concentrations as assessed by T2-MRI where approximately 14% of patients with cardiac iron overload were identified who had no matched degree of hepatic hemosiderosis [24].

6.3. Molecular genetic analysis

PCR-based procedures can detect the commonly occurring mutations in β-globin gene. The most commonly used methods are reverse dot blot analysis or primer-specific amplification, with a set of probes complementary to the most common mutations in each population. β-Globin gene sequence analysis is used to detect mutations in the β-globin gene in case of failure of targeted mutation analysis [25].

6.4. Prenatal diagnosis

Prenatal diagnosis is possible through analysis of DNA obtained through chorionic villi sampling at 8–10 weeks' fetal gestation or by amniocentesis at 14–20 weeks' gestation. In most laboratories, the DNA is amplified using the PCR assay test and then is analyzed for the presence of the thalassemia mutation using a panel of oligonucleotide probes corresponding to known thalassemia mutations. Prenatal diagnosis may be performed noninvasively, with the use of maternal blood samples to isolate either fetal cells or fetal DNA for analysis [26].

7. Treatment of thalassemia

7.1. Transfusion therapy

In general, children with β-thalassemia major and hemoglobins of less than 6–7 g/dl should receive chronic transfusions. It is important to start early before the child has a chance to develop splenomegaly and hypersplenism and before skeletal changes and growth retardation. It is also important to establish a reliable, routine transfusion schedule that maintains hemoglobin levels of 9–10 g/dl [27].

Transfusions of washed, leukocyte-depleted RBCs are recommended for all the patients to reduce the incidence of febrile and urticarial reactions as well as infectious cytomegalovirus contamination [28]. Extended red cell antigen typing, including at least the Rh antigens, Duffy, Kidd, and Kell, is recommended before the patient is started on a transfusion regimen [27].

7.2. Iron chelation therapy

Children with thalassemia major should begin therapy at the earliest possible age and certainly by the time they have accumulated more than 7 g of excess iron. In young children, a serum ferritin level much greater than 1.000 µg/l or 1 year of regular transfusions (or both) can be used as surrogate indicators to initiate chelation therapy [27].

7.2.1. Deferoxamine

Deferoxamine (DFO) is a hexadentate iron chelator (deferoxamine mesylate; desferal®). DFO was introduced as parenteral therapy for iron overload associated with β-thalassemia major in 1976 [30]. Plasma half-life of DFO is short (20–30 min). Therefore, standard treatment involves the subcutaneous infusion of 40 mg DFO for 8–12 h nightly for 5–7 nights weekly using a battery-operated infusion pump. Subcutaneous administration is preferred except in patients with severe cardiac iron deposition, for whom continuous intravenous deferoxamine therapy is recommended. Iron excretion occurs through biliary and urinary routes [29].

Adverse events of DFO include growth retardation, skeletal changes, ocular and auditory disturbances, pulmonary, and renal toxicities. They are preventable if proper monitoring is practiced to detect early signs of toxicity. Susceptibility to infection with Yersinia and perhaps other Gram-negative bacilli is increased in thalassemia patients who receive DFO therapy. Painful local skin reactions at the infusion site are common. Zinc deficiency can occur [29].

7.2.2. Deferiprone

Deferiprone (DFP) is an orally administered bidentate iron chelator (Ferriprox®, Kelfer®). The usual dose of DFP is 75–100 mg/kg/day taken orally in three divided doses. Plasma half-life of DFP is 2–3 h, and iron is mainly excreted in urine [30]. Adverse effects of DFP include gastrointestinal disturbances, agranulocytosis and neutropenia, arthropathy, increased liver enzyme levels, and low plasma zinc level [29, 30].

7.2.3. Deferasirox

Deferasirox (DFX) is an orally administered tridentate iron chelator that is indicated for the treatment of transfusion iron overload in persons more than 2 years of age. The US Food and Drug Administration approves a recommended daily dose of 20–40 mg/kg body weight, taken once on an empty stomach at least 30 min before food [29]. The most common adverse events with DFX therapy include gastrointestinal disturbances, rash, and mild increases in serum creatinine [31].

7.2.4. Combination therapy

1. "Shuttle hypothesis": combination of DFO and deferiprone

Combined DFO and DFP regimens offer an alternative option for patients with severe heart disease. Deferiprone, though a weaker chelator, is a relatively small uncharged molecule that can enter the cardiac cells more easily than DFO and transfers the chelated iron from the myocardial cells to the stronger chelator, DFO in the plasma [32].

2. Combination of Deferasirox and DFO

The efficacy of combining DFO with Deferasirox has been assessed in a number of studies. This combination has an additive effect, allows decreasing the dose of both chelators and improves the compliance. The "shuttle effect" is also applicable with this combination as Deferasirox acts as an intracellular chelator and DFO as a powerful extracellular chelator [32].

7.3. Splenectomy

Splenectomy is recommended when the calculated annual transfusion requirement is >200 to 220 ml RBCs/kg per year with a hematocrit of 70%. Splenectomy may be necessary to decrease the disabling effects of abdominal pressure and to increase the life span of supplemental RBCs. After splenectomy, children generally require fewer transfusions, although the basic defect in Hb synthesis remains unaffected. Splenectomy is a therapy that should not be considered casually because susceptibility to infection with *Streptococcus pneumoniae, Haemophilus influenza,* and *Neisseria meningitids* increases after splenectomy in children, particularly in those younger than 5 years. Standard therapy for splenectomized individuals includes immunizations, prophylactic penicillin, and a high index of suspicion and aggressive antibiotic therapy for febrile illness. Thromboembolic events and pulmonary hypertension are also increased in splenectomized patients. These complications may be minimized by the routine use of aspirin or low dose anticoagulants [28].

7.4. Stem cell transplantation (SCT)

SCT or bone marrow transplantation (BMT) is the only possible, proven curative treatment for β-thalassemia major. The most important role of SCT is the high chance of cure for individuals who otherwise face a lifetime of invasive, demanding treatment and a reduced life span [33].

7.5. Vitamin supplementation

Vitamin E supplementation in thalassemia major is often suggested, but data demonstrating its efficacy are lacking. Folic acid supplements help to maintain folic acid levels in the face of increased requirements [27].

7.6. Fetal hemoglobin induction

In β-thalassemia, pharmacologically induced increase in γ-globin chains would be expected to decrease globin chain imbalance with consequent amelioration of clinical manifestation. Pharmacologically, three classes of agents have been shown to be capable of inducing HbF to therapeutic levels: erythropoietins, short-chain fatty acid derivatives, and chemotherapeutic agents. Hydroxyurea has been recommended in patients with thalassemia intermedia [28].

7.7. Gene therapy

B-Thalassemia is a potential attractive target for gene therapy. This could be a reality if a functional β-globin gene could be safely and efficiently introduced into the hematopoietic stem cells, and lineage-restricted expression of the β-globin protein exceeding 15% could be achieved in erythroid progenitor cells. Gene therapy for β-thalassemia requires gene transfer into hematopoietic stem cells (HSCs) using integrating vectors that direct the regulated expression of β-globin at therapeutic levels [34].

8. Prevention

Prevention strategies include community education, carrier detection, genetic counseling, and prenatal diagnosis [27].

9. Conclusion

β-Thalassemias are markedly heterogeneous at their molecular level with a clear association between genotype and clinical phenotype. Study of the molecular genetics in patients with β-thalassemia in their early life will serve as a tool to predict clinical disease severity and help in planning of early intervention strategies.

Author details

Tamer Hassan*, Mohamed Badr, Usama El Safy, Mervat Hesham, Laila Sherief and Marwa Zakaria

*Address all correspondence to: dr.tamerhassan@yahoo.com

Department of Pediatrics, Zagazig University, Egypt

References

[1] Flint J, Harding RM, Boyce AJ, Clegg JB. The population genetics of the haemoglobinopathies. Bailliere's Clin Hematol. 1998;11(1):1–51. DOI: 10.1016/S0950-3536(98)80069-3

[2] Vichinsky EP. Changing patterns of thalassemia worldwide. Ann N Y Acad Sci. 2005;1054(1):18–24. DOI: 10.1196/annals.1345.003

[3] El-Beshlawy A, Kaddah N, Rageb L, Hussein I, Mouktar G, Moustafa A, Elraouf E, Hassaballa N, T Gaafar and El-Sendiony H. Thalassemia prevalence and status in Egypt. Pediatric Res. 1999;45(S5):760. DOI: 10.1203/00006450-199905010-00132

[4] Giardine B, van Baal S, Kaimakis P, Riemer C, Miller W, Samara M, Kollia P, Anagnou NP, Chui DH, Wajcman H, Hardison RC, Patrinos GP. HbVar database of human hemoglobin variants and thalassemia mutations: 2007 update. Hum Mutat. 2007;28(2): 206–206. DOI: 10.1002/humu.9479

[5] Ward AJ, Cooper TA. The pathobiology of splicing. J Pathol. 2010;220(2):152–163. DOI: 10.1002/path.2649

[6] Galanello R, Cao A. Relationship between genotype and phenotype. Thalassemia intermedia. Ann N Y Acad Sci. 1998;850(1):325–333. DOI: 10.1111/j.1749-6632.1998.tb10489.x

[7] Origa R, Galanello R, Perseu L, Tavazzi D, Domenica Cappellini M, Terenzani L, Forni GL, Quarta G, Boetti T, Piga A. Cholelithiasis in thalassemia major. Eur J Haematol. 2009;82(1):22–25. DOI: 10.1111/j.1600-0609.2008.01162.x

[8] Economou-Petersen E, Aessopos A, Kladi A, Flevari P, Karabatsos F, Fragodimitri C, Nicolaidis P, Vrettou H, Vassilopoulos D, Karagiorga-Lagana M, Kremastinos DT, Petersen MB. Apolipoprotein E epsilon4 allele as a genetic risk factor for left ventricular failure in homozygous beta-thalassemia. Blood. 1998;92(9):3455–3459. DOI: http://dx.doi.org/

[9] Longo F, Zecchina G, Sbaiz L, Fischer R, Piga A, Camaschella C. The influence of hemochromatosis mutations on iron overload of thalassemia major. Haematologica. 1999;84(9):799–803.

[10] Origa R, Satta S, Matta G, Galanello R. Glutathione S-transferase gene polymorphism and cardiac iron overload in thalassemia major. Br J Haematol. 2008;142(1):143–145. DOI: 10.1111/j.1365-2141.2008.07175.x

[11] Sollaino MC, Paglietti ME, Perseu L, Giagu N, Loi D, Galanello R. Association of alpha globin gene quadruplication and heterozygous beta thalassemia in patients with thalassemia intermedia. Haematologica. 2009;94(10):1445–1448. DOI: 10.3324/haematol.2009.005728

[12]   Schrier SL. Pathophysiology of thalassemia. Curr Opin Hematol. 2002;9(2):123–126.

[13]   Rivella S. the role of ineffective erythropoiesis in non-transfusion-dependent thalasse-mia. Blood Rev. 2012;26(1):S12–S15. DOI: 10.1016/S0268-960X(12)70005-X

[14]   Grinberg LN, Rachmilewitz EA, Kitrossky N, Chevion M. Hydroxyl radical generation in beta-thalassemic red blood cells. Free Radic Biol Med. 1995;18(3):611–615. DOI: 10.1016/0891-5849(94)00160-L

[15]   Nienhuis AW, Nathan DG. Pathophysiology and clinical manifestations of the β-thalassemias. Cold Spring Harb Perspect Med. 2012;2(12):a011726. DOI: 10.1101/cshperspect.a011726

[16]   Cunningham MJ, Macklin EA, Neufeld EJ, Cohen AR; Thalassemia Clinical Research Network. Complications of beta-thalassemia major in North America. Blood. 2004;104(1):34–39. http:10.1182/blood-2003-09-3167.

[17]   Jacobs EM, Hendriks JC, van Tits BL, Evans PJ, Breuer W, Liu DY, et al. Results of an international round robin for the quantification of serum non-transferrin-bound iron: Need for defining standardization and a clinically relevant isoform. Anal Biochem. 2005;341(2):241–250. DOI: 10.1016/j.ab.2005.03.008

[18]   Pootrakul P, Breuer W, Sametband M, Sirankapracha P, Hershko C, Cabantchik ZI. Labile plasma iron (LPI) as an indicator of chelatable plasma redox activity in iron-overloaded beta-thalassemia/HbE patients treated with an oral chelator. Blood. 2004;104(5):1504–1510. DOI: http:10.1182/blood-2004-02-0630

[19]   Kemna EH, Tjalsma H, Podust VN, Swinkels DW. Mass spectrometry-based hepcidin measurements in serum and urine: analytical aspects and clinical implications. Clin Chem. 2007;53(4):620–628. DOI: 10.1373/clinchem.2006.079186

[20]   Beutler E, Hoffbrand AV, Cook JD. Iron deficiency and overload. Hematology (Am Soc Hematol Educ Program). 2003;2003(1):40–61. DOI: 10.1182/asheducation-2003.1.40

[21]   Fucharoen S, Ketvichit P, Pootrakul P, Siritanaratkul N, Piankijagum A, Wasi P. Clinical manifestation of beta-thalassemia/hemoglobin E disease. J Pediatr Hematol Oncol. 2000;22(6):552–557. DOI: 00043426-200011000-00022

[22]   Galanello R, Kattamis A, Piga A, Fischer R, Leoni G, Ladis V, Voi V, et al. A prospective randomized controlled trial on the safety and efficacy of alternating desferrioxamine and deferiprone in the treatment of iron overload in patients with thalassemia. Haematologica. 2006;91(9):1241–1243.

[23]   Hankins JS, McCarville MB, Loeffler RB, Smeltzer MP, Onciu M, Hoffer FA, et al. R2* magnetic resonance imaging of the liver in patients with iron overload. Blood. 2009;113(20):4853–4855. DOI: 10.1182/blood-2008-12-191643

[24]   Deborah Chirnomas S, Geukes-Foppen M, Barry K, Braunstein J, Kalish LA, Neufeld EJ, et al. Practical implications of liver and heart iron load assessment by T2*-MRI in

children and adults with transfusion-dependent anemias. Am J Hematol. 2008;83(10): 781–783. DOI: 10.1002/ajh.21221

[25] Galanello R, Origa R. Beta-thalassemia. Orphanet J Rare Dis. 2010;5(11)DOI: doi: 10.1186/1750-1172-5-11

[26] Colah RB, Gorakshakar AC, Nadkarni AH. Invasive & non-invasive approaches for prenatal diagnosis of haemoglobinopathies: experiences from India. Indian J Med Res. 2011;134(4):552–560.

[27] Borgna-Pignatti C, Galanello R. Thalassemias and related disorders: Quantitative disorders of hemoglobin synthesis. In: Greer JP, Foerster J, Rodger GM, Paraskevas F, Glader B, Means RT, editors. Wintrobe's Clinical Hematology. 12th ed. Philadelphia: Lippincott Williams and Wilkins; 2009. p. 1082–1131.

[28] Rachmilewitz EA, Giardina PJ. How I treat thalassemia. Blood. 2011;118(13):3479–3488. DOI: 10.1182/blood-2010-08-300335

[29] Barton JC, Edwards CQ, Phatak PD, Britton RS, Bacon BR. Handbook of Iron Overload Disorders. 1st ed. Cambridge: Cambridge University Press; 2010. 386 p.

[30] Brittenham GM. Iron-chelating therapy for transfusional iron overload. N Engl J Med. 2011;364(2):146–156. DOI: 10.1056/NEJMct1004810

[31] Berdoukas V, Chouliaras G, Moraitis P, Zannikos K, Berdoussi E, Ladis V. The efficacy of iron chelator regimes in reducing cardiac and hepatic iron in patients with thalas-saemia major: a clinical observational study. J Cardiovasc Magn Reson. 2009;11(20):1–11. DOI: doi: 10.1186/1532-429X-11-20

[32] Prabhu R, Prabhu V, Prabhu RS. iron overload in beta thalassemia – a review. J Biosci Tech. 2009;1(1):21–30.

[33] Bhatia M, Walters MC. Hematopoietic cell transplantation for thalassemia and sickle cell disease: past, present and future. Bone Marrow Transplant. 2008;41(2):109–117.

[34] Rivers AE, Srivastava A. Gene therapy of hemoglobinopathies. In: Herzog RW, Zolotukhin S, editors. A Guide to Human Gene Therapy. 1st ed. Singapore: World Scientific Publishing Co.; 2010. p. 197–199.